THE JUICING RECIPES BOOK

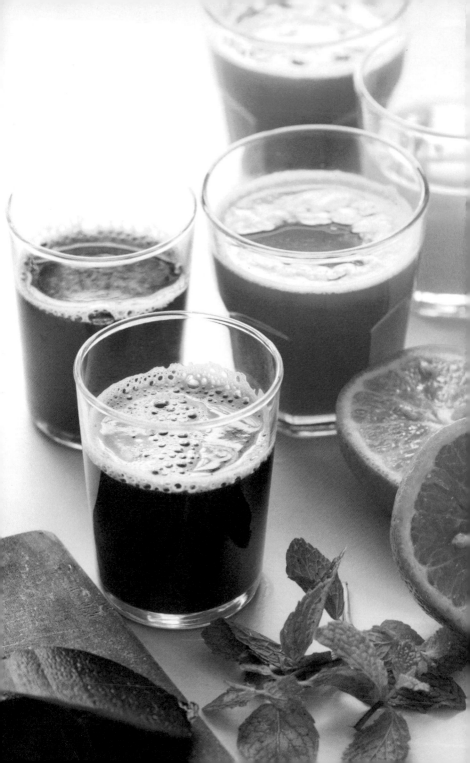

THE
JUICING
RECIPES
BOOK

150
HEALTHY JUICING RECIPES
TO UNLEASH THE NUTRITIONAL POWER
OF YOUR JUICER MACHINE

MENDOCINO
PRESS

CONTENTS

INTRODUCTION

Welcome to the world of juicing! Perhaps you've become curious about juicing because of a health care practitioner's suggestion, or at the recommendation of a friend. Perhaps you heard about it on TV, saw it in a magazine, or read it on a late-night Internet binge. Whatever way you've discovered juicing, congratulations! Juicing is one of the best ways to enhance your health, for good reason. Convenient, easy, and fun, juicing fresh fruits and vegetables optimizes your intake of essential vitamins, minerals, and other nutrients, without the fuss of preparing elaborate meals. Proven to help kick-start your metabolism, boost your mood, and nourish your brain, juicing can help you achieve your nutrition goals or enhance an already healthy lifestyle. Freshly made juices are packed with powerful disease-fighting antioxidants and phytochemicals in a readily accessible and delicious form.

You can often infer how nutritious and antioxidant-packed a fruit or vegetable is by looking at the color—if it sports greens, reds, oranges, or other bright colors, it is most likely high in nutrition and ideal for juicing. Some of the recipes in this book—such as Orange-Cranberry or Grapefruit, Carrot, and Ginger—are simply nutritious and tasty ways to start your day. Others have more specific health goals in mind, such as Watermelon-Mint to aid digestive health, or Tomato Tonic to combat the aging process.

Chapters 1 and 2 will introduce you to the different types of juicers and how to select one that's right for you, as well as common juicing ingredients and how to prep them for best results. Starting with Chapter 3, the recipes are organized into categories based on the juice's properties. Each juice recipe includes nutritional information and can be made using just a few, readily available ingredients. Additionally, recipes are coded by their suitability for the three different types of juicers discussed in Chapter 1, using handy icons.

One thing to remember is that many of the juices in this book fit into multiple categories; for example, most green juices are also great for cleanses and weight loss. With that in mind, the following list is a preview of each recipe category, and the expected health benefits therein. You'll soon discover your favorites, and you can flip back to this list anytime you feel like experimenting or want a quick reminder of what juices to use for specific purposes.

- *Breakfast Juices:* Chapter 3 is packed with great-tasting juices to start the day. Flavor, availability of ingredients, and breakfast nutrition goals are prioritized in this chapter. Almost all the juices in this book are excellent breakfast choices, but Chapter 7 (Antioxidant Juices), Chapter 11 (High-Energy Juices), and Chapter 14 (Kid-Friendly Juices) are particularly good places to look.

- *Brain-Nourishing Juices:* Chapter 4 focuses on ingredients such as cucumber, blueberries, and spinach, all of which can contribute to improved mental health. These juices can help alleviate stress and depression, improve sleep and memory, and generally help your brain stay healthy.

- *Alkalizing Juices:* Some research hints that a diet low in acid-producing foods—like animal proteins, refined sugar, and bread—and high in fruits and veggies may help prevent kidney stones, improve cardiovascular health, reduce muscle and joint pain, and lower risk for certain diseases. All of the recipes found in Chapter 5 support an alkaline diet plan.

- *Anti-Aging Juices:* Whether you are looking to prevent or reduce wrinkles, relieve the symptoms of menopause, or reset your metabolism, Chapter 6 is for you.

- *Antioxidant Juices:* Antioxidants are the vitamins and nutrients the body needs to neutralize free radicals, which are known to cause a wide array of health problems. Antioxidants have been shown to slow the aging process and may help prevent certain diseases, including cancers. All the juices in Chapter 7 are especially high in these compounds.

- *Cleansing Juices:* Many cleansing diets have sprung up in recent years, several of which "conveniently" come paired with processed, high-cost juices. Chapter 8 offers body-cleansing juices you can make on your own to save money while also getting nutritional benefits. Pair these juices with those in Chapter 10 for an extra cleansing boost.

- *Diabetic-Friendly Juices:* The recipes in Chapter 9, such as Essential Mineral Infusion and Vitamin E Veggie Supplement, emphasize ingredients that help maintain proper insulin levels and prevent spikes in blood sugar. In addition to the basic nutritional information provided for each recipe, make sure to discuss your nutritional needs with your doctor to decide what juices in other chapters may also be great additions to your diet.

- *Digestive Health Juices:* The juices in Chapter 10 focus on digestive health, including cures for common ailments like bloating, gas, indigestion, sour stomach, and intestinal pain. For example, a Pineapple and Pear Cooler fortified with mint leaves makes a great overall tonic for digestive relief and health. As is true with any change in diet directed at treating a health ailment, consult a physician if symptoms persist or get worse.

- *High-Energy Juices:* Nearly any juice in this book will give your energy levels a kick into high gear. However, the juices in Chapter 11 are especially tailored to increase your metabolism, improve your sleep, and provide a caffeine-free boost to your day. Wake up your system with The Cure for What Kales You, or down a shot of Energy Boost made with wheatgrass and cranberries for a midday pick-me-up.

- *Green Juices:* Incorporating green vegetables into a juice is a great way to reduce calories and sugars while providing an infusion of added nutrients. Chapter 12 describes some of the most common green juices, formulated to be refreshing, tasty, and easy to make. (You will find other examples of green juices throughout the book, but they are especially common in Chapter 5 and Chapter 8.)

- *Healthful Skin Juices:* Nutrition and hydration play a major role in skin health, so it's no wonder juices are a popular way to fortify your skin with the essential vitamins and minerals needed for a bright and acne-free complexion. In Chapter 13, you'll want to try Papaya Power for wrinkle prevention, or treat yourself to a Skin-Strengthening Antioxidant Blast made with equal parts yellow beets, blackberries, and strawberries.

- *Kid-Friendly Juices:* It's no secret that kids love juice. However, the heavily processed and often artificially sweetened juices occupying store shelves leave much to be desired when seeking healthy treats. The juices in Chapter 14 are tailored to tickle your tot's taste buds, and also sneak in just enough veggies to lower the sugar count and increase nutrition without sacrificing flavor.

- *Low-Fat Juices:* All the juices found in Chapter 15 contain 1 gram of fat or less without skimping on flavor. Sweet Potato and Spice makes a truly tempting drinkable dessert, and Cinnamon Fat Control adds a burst of flavor while helping regulate blood sugar levels.

- *Protein Juices:* How to get enough protein when juicing is a common question for the uninitiated. All the juices in Chapter 16 contain at least 5 grams of protein. The protein content of juices are also listed throughout the book, and you will quickly notice that a good number of juices get at least 10 percent of their calories from protein.

- *Weight-Loss Juices:* The juices in Chapter 17 go beyond low calorie counts. These recipes also feature ingredients known to boost metabolism, pair well with exercise routines, and suppress appetite. Choose Pineapple,

Cucumber, and Romaine for a great meal replacement juice that will also satisfy a sweet tooth, or drink your salad with Vegetable Weight-Loss Juice, which will help keep you feeling energized and full.

Whether you want to try juicing to lose weight, cleanse your body of toxins, manage your mental health, or simply enjoy a refreshing and healthy alternative to store-bought beverages, this book will get you started. With 151 recipes to sample, plus tips along the way for choosing and using fresh, flavorful ingredients, you'll be a juicing pro in no time. Happy juicing!

Understanding the nutritional content of your freshly made juice. The nutritional information listed for each recipe is meant only as a guide. Your actual results will vary depending on the size, quality, and type of ingredients you use and the kind of juicer you have. The nutritional information provided corresponds to the average you can expect, and each recipe makes a single serving.

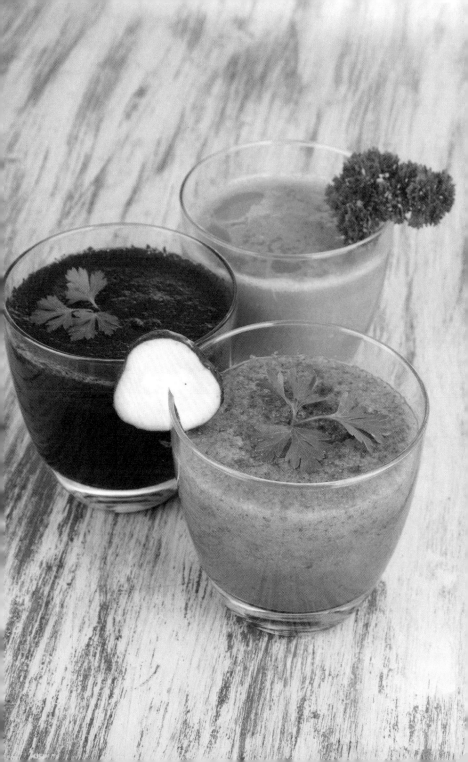

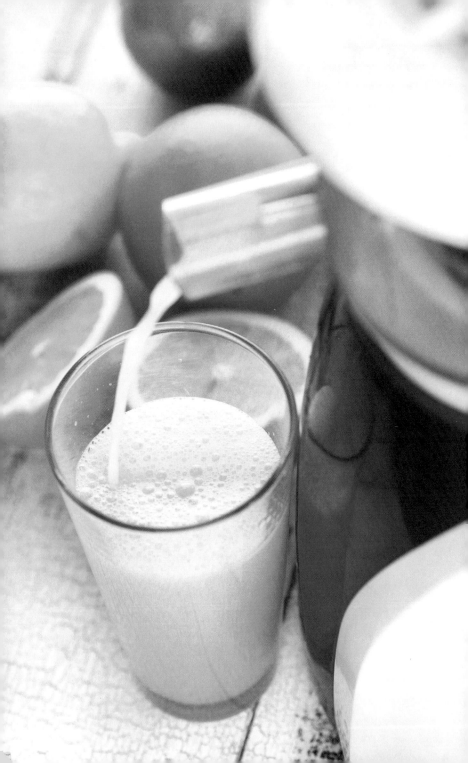

1

KNOW
YOUR
JUICER

A juicer is a mechanical device that processes produce, separating the nutrient-rich liquids from the fibrous pulp. There are numerous juicers and categories of juicers on the market these days, but there is no need to feel daunted by the multitude of choices. Once you become familiar with the three main types of juicers, it will be much easier to select one that suits your preferences and your budget.

Cost can be a big factor in choosing a juicer. If you plan on doing a lot of juicing, it is wise to consider how efficient your juicer is. Saving money up front on a less-productive model may result in spending even more money on produce over the years. While a whole spectrum of juicers exists, it does pay to invest in the juicer that's best for your long-term purposes. This chapter describes each of the major types of juicers, while detailing features to consider as you decide which one is right for you. Look for the icons on each recipe page to know which type(s) of juicers will work best for the recipe.

TYPES OF JUICERS

ⓒ CENTRIFUGAL JUICER

A centrifugal juicer is the most common type of juicing device. It is one of the oldest types of electric juicers, and one of the cheapest varieties available on the market. This device uses spinning blades to pulverize the produce, coupled with a spinning fine-mesh strainer that separates the juice from the pulp.

Most centrifugal juicers dump the pulp into a separate container, allowing you to process a large amount of fruits and vegetables without stopping. Besides being one of the least expensive options, centrifugal juicers also tend to be one of the fastest and easiest to operate. Not only do they process produce quickly, but their feed tube is usually big enough to allow a whole fruit—or at least very large chunks of it—to go through without the need for chopping. Look for a model that has removable parts that are easy to clean (or, better yet, dishwasher safe).

Centrifugal juicers do have a few drawbacks. Because the mechanism behind the juicer spins so fast, it produces a fair amount of heat, which can reduce the nutritional content of your juice. Using well-refrigerated produce can help minimize this damage. Centrifugal juicers also tend to be more wasteful than other types—in some cases yielding less than half the juice of the others. They do a particularly poor job with leafy greens.

Finally, the high-speed spinning action of centrifugal juicers produces a large amount of froth and oxygenates the final product. Oxygen does two things to your juice: First, it actually enhances the flavor, similar to decanting wine in order to allow it to "breathe" a bit before drinking it. The downside

Getting some leafy green nutrition with a centrifugal juicer. If you want to incorporate the occasional leafy green using this type of juicer, follow these simple tricks: For larger leaves like kale and large-leaf spinach, you can roll up the leaves as you would a newspaper and add them to the juicer. You can also sandwich smaller leaves between fleshier fruits and feed them through the juicer this way. Another option, especially with delicate greens such as baby spinach, is to juice everything but the greens, and then process the juice and greens in a blender until smooth. Doing this allows you to use about half the greens to get the same nutritional benefit—as well as some added fiber!

is that oxygen also oxidizes the nutrients and other components of the juice, reducing its nutritional value. Additionally, high oxygen levels will cause juices to spoil more quickly. In general, it is advisable to drink juice made from these types of juicers the same day you make it.

If you are looking for a simple, entry-level juicer, are often in a hurry, or plan on mostly juicing fruits, root vegetables, and other fleshy veggies, then a centrifugal juicer may be a good choice for you.

Ⓜ MASTICATING JUICER

Masticating juicers were designed to avoid the limitations of centrifugal juicers. In these types of juicers, the produce is manually crushed and squeezed, extracting a much higher yield of juice without added heat or oxygenation. Masticating juicers squeeze pulp until it is dry, making them a great choice for leafy greens as well as for fleshier fruits and vegetables.

Because they do such a great job of squeezing out juice, you will want to at least partially peel lemons and limes before using these juicers. Otherwise, you will end up with a rather bitter-tasting juice. Most masticating juicers require the produce fed into them to be cut up into small pieces, adding some prep work to your juicing. These juicers also tend to be louder, more expensive, and somewhat slower than centrifugal juicers. The components can also be more complicated, making cleanup a bit more time-consuming.

Juices made from masticating juicers tend to keep longer, staying fresh for up to 3 days, depending on the ingredients used. If you don't mind a little extra effort to improve nutritional yield, you may want to consider investing in a masticating juicer.

ⓣ TRITURATING JUICER

Triturating juicers are incredibly efficient machines, excelling at extracting juice from fruits and vegetables. Unlike the other machines mentioned, triturating juicers use multiple mechanisms to extract juice. This allows them to have the highest

Maintaining and cleaning your juicer. To extend the life of your juicer, always keep it clean and in proper working order. That little bit of wet pulp might seem inconsequential, but it can dry with gluelike properties and interfere with the operation of your juicer. Before you start juicing, check that all the components are clean and properly in place to avoid risk of injury. Be sure to read your juicer's instruction manual to understand how to operate it correctly.

Tips for juicing citrus. All the juicers mentioned in this chapter will do at least a passable job on citrus fruits. However, none can really compare to the convenience and yield of a cheap citrus juicer, which also lets you skip peeling. If you find yourself gravitating toward juices that involve a lot of these vitamin C—packed fruits, you might want to consider getting a basic citrus juicer to juice them separately before combining them with other ingredients.

yield of any juicer on the market, but also means that they are slower and have even more moving parts to clean. Their feed tubes also tend to be smaller, requiring more prep work. These juicers are generally the most expensive, often costing several hundred dollars for a quality machine.

Triturating juicers are multifunctional. In addition to juice, they can make nut butters, frozen desserts, pasta, and even baby food using the various accessories that come with the machines. In other words, a triturating juicer can work as a food processor as well, helping defray the initial cost. The only produce they do not process well are citrus fruits, though they still do an acceptable job in most cases. Because the juicer extracts nearly every drop of liquid from your produce, take care to remove seeds and peels that may impart bitter flavors.

If your goal is to obtain the absolute maximum amount of juice at the highest quality, and if the investment in the machinery and time it requires are less of a concern for you, then this category of juicer might be worth exploring.

Use this chart as a quick reference for choosing which juicer to buy and what recipes to start with if you already own a particular model. You will find plenty of recipes in each juicing category to use with your juicer.

Type of Juicer	Method	Cost	Required Food Prep	Best Suited for
CENTRIFUGAL Ⓒ	Pulverizes	Lower cost	Minimal chopping	Fruits, root vegetables, and fleshy vegetables
MASTICATING Ⓜ	Crushes/ squeezes	Moderate cost	Peeling and chopping	Leafy greens, fleshy fruits and vegetables
TRITURATING Ⓣ	Uses multiple mechanisms	High cost	Fine chopping	Fruits, vegetables, and much more

A note about grapefruit juice. *Grapefruit juice blocks an enzyme in the intestine that normally slows the absorption of many medications. Mixing grapefruit and medications can be hazardous, so be sure to check labels and ask your health care provider about any prescribed medications you are taking.*

JUICING ACCESSORIES

Once you've decided which type of juicer to buy, a few handy kitchen tools (some of which you may already have) will make everyday juicing a cinch:

- Paring knife and cutting board

- Vegetable peeler

- Blender (for incorporating bananas or other ingredients that can't be juiced)

- Potato scrubber or other stiff-bristled brush (for cleaning especially dirty root vegetables or fruits with deep ridges, like pineapples)

- Measuring cups, spatulas, and stirring spoons

- Food scale (to carefully monitor ingredients)

- Dish brush (for removing stubborn pulp when cleaning the juicer)

- Compost bin (to make productive use of the waste)

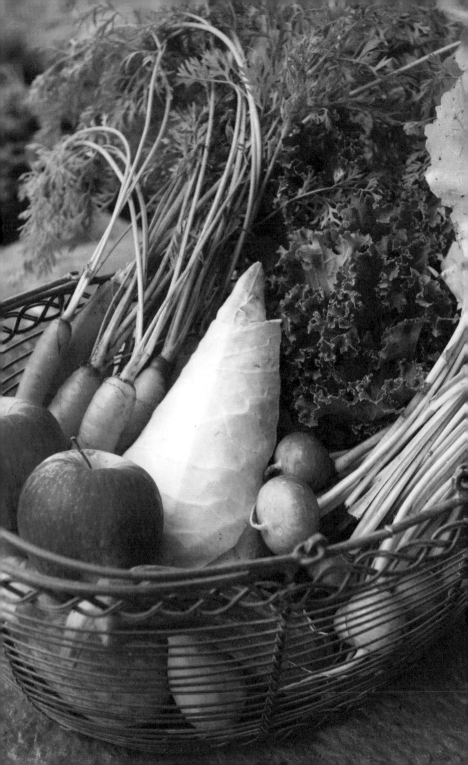

2

JUICING
INGREDIENTS

This chapter will acquaint you with some of the most common juicing ingredients and how best to store and use them so that you can begin juicing with confidence and ease. For the most healthful results, seek out produce that is as local as possible and organic. Farm or CSA (community-supported agriculture) shares, which are growing in popularity across the country, are a great way to get a constant and plentiful supply of local produce that is usually grown following organic practices.

Unfortunately, in most areas it is impossible to locate a source of fresh, local, and organic produce year-round. Even in winter months, though, you may be able to find a great selection; choose wisely, and if you must buy nonorganic fruits and vegetables, make sure to wash and/or peel them to avoid ingesting unwanted chemicals.

While frozen fruit, once thawed, can be juiced relatively well, it still makes a bit of a mess, and many juicers have trouble getting a good yield. Never try to juice any canned or jarred fruit, as it's often heat pasteurized and packed with syrup.

JUICING INGREDIENTS
TO KEEP ON HAND

Stocking a few key items will allow you to make an impromptu juice whenever the urge strikes. The following ingredients are some of the most commonly used when juicing. The list also includes information on how to store the produce properly so it will last. Once you have cut into any piece of produce, it should be enclosed in an airtight container and stored in the refrigerator, preferably for use as soon as possible.

- *Apples:* Store in the refrigerator or a root cellar. Apples should be stored separately from other produce, as their skin emits a gas that quickens the ripening process.

- *Beets:* Store in a root cellar (without greens) or refrigerator. Use greens within a few days, before they wilt.

- *Carrots:* Store in the refrigerator for up to 1 month.

- *Celery:* Store in the refrigerator for up to 2 weeks, but use within 1 week if making use of the delicate greens.

- *Citrus:* Store at room temperature. Storing in the refrigerator will add some time to its shelf life, but do not store citrus in a plastic bag or in close contact with other produce.

- *Ginger:* Refrigerating this rhizome will extend its life to several weeks or months. Wrap loosely in a plastic bag, and use only while still firm to the touch.

- *Grapes:* Store in the refrigerator.

- *Kale and other leafy greens:* Wrap loosely in a plastic bag, and keep in the crisper of your refrigerator.

- *Melons:* Store in a cool, dry place for several days or weeks.

- *Pineapples:* These do not ripen once picked and should be juiced as soon as possible to maximize nutrition. Pineapples can be stored for up to 5 days in the refrigerator.

- *Tomatoes:* Store in a cool, dark place.

HOW TO PREP FRUITS AND VEGETABLES FOR JUICING

Generally, prepping produce for juicing is pretty easy. With a few exceptions, the peels and seeds can go right in as well—the juicer will filter them out along with the pulp, even extracting some nutrients along the way. Follow the general guidelines listed here, and consult the Produce Prep Chart on page 21 for more detailed instructions for individual ingredients.

Always wash fruits and vegetables thoroughly before juicing. Root vegetables; produce with large pits or crevices in the skin, such as pineapple and cantaloupe; and nonorganic or waxed produce generally require some scrubbing with a stiff-bristled brush.

Check your juicer's manual for the proper size to cut. Centrifugal juicers generally can handle anything that will fit in the feed tube. Masticating and triturating juicers usually require produce to be chopped into more manageable pieces.

The skins of oranges and grapefruit contain essential oils that can cause severe stomach discomfort. Leaving some of the white pith after peeling is fine, though—in fact, it will actually add more nutrients into your juice. Lemons and limes can generally be juiced whole or partially peeled, depending on the type of juicer you have. Check your juicer's manual for guidelines on peeling and seeding.

Always remove stony pits or seeds such as those found in plums, cherries, peaches, mangos, and apricots.

Similarly, remove any woody stems, such as the thicker stems of grapes, which can dull or even break the blades of your juicer. Smaller bits of stems like those found on apples or strawberries are fine.

Cut out any bruises, blemishes, and brown spots.

What not to juice. *Bananas, avocados, nuts, coconuts, and other oily or low-water produce should never be put in a juicer—they simply mash up. Instructions for how to incorporate these ingredients are detailed in the recipes in this book. Strawberries, papayas, and cantaloupes don't let go of their juice very well. In this book, the amounts required of these ingredients are adjusted accordingly so they can be juiced along with everything else, but you can also cut their amounts in half and process with the rest of the juice in a blender to make a more smoothielike beverage.*

PRODUCE PREP CHART

Produce Variety	Preparation Instructions
Alfalfa sprouts	Wash thoroughly and pat dry.
Apples, all varieties	Rinse and remove any leaves on the stem. While the seeds contain trace levels of an organic cyanide compound, the human body is able to metabolize far greater quantities than the seeds will ever provide.
Asparagus	Wash thoroughly and trim the woody ends.
Bananas	Do not put bananas in any juicer. To add banana, peel and combine with fresh juice in a blender and process until smooth. Always use a very ripe banana for best results.
Basil	Wash thoroughly and pat dry. Trim the ends of the stems and remove any blemished leaves.
Bean sprouts	Wash thoroughly and pat dry.
Beets, red or yellow	Peel skin or scrub thoroughly. Rinse the greens thoroughly, trimming any brown spots.
Bell peppers, all colors	Rinse thoroughly and remove the woody stems. Remove the seeds and white inner pith for a less bitter juice (optional).
Blackberries	Rinse.
Blueberries	Rinse.
Broccoli	Rinse and trim the ends of the stems.
Brussels sprouts	Rinse and remove any spots. Remove the stalks.
Cabbage, green or red	Remove the tough outer leaves. ➤

Produce Variety	Preparation Instructions
Cantaloupe	Scrub, slice into 1-inch-thick wedges (or whatever size will fit in your juicer's feed tube), and remove the seeds. For masticating juicers, remove the peels and seeds; then chop to the size recommended by your juicer's instructions.
Carrots	Scrub thoroughly or peel. Remove the green tops and any dark spots.
Cauliflower	Rinse and cut off the ends of the stems.
Celery	Rinse and remove the root base. Include the leaves unless you want a milder flavor.
Cherries, all types	Rinse and remove the pits.
Cilantro	Rinse thoroughly and pat dry. Trim the ends of the stems and remove any blemished leaves.
Collard greens	Rinse thoroughly and remove any brown spots.
Cranberries	Rinse.
Cucumbers	If unwaxed, rinse. If waxed, peel or scrub thoroughly. You can leave the seeds in for added liquid and nutrition, but the seeds can add some bitterness to the juice, so remove if desired.
Endive	Rinse and remove the tough outer layers.
Fennel	Rinse and trim the ends.
Garlic	Peel off the papery outer layers.
Ginger	Scrub clean. Leave the skin intact.
Grapefruits	Peel and cut into a size appropriate to fit in your juicer.

Grapes, all varieties	Remove the stems and rinse.
Green beans	Rinse.
Honeydew melon	Scrub, slice into 1-inch-thick wedges (or whatever size will fit in your juicer's feed tube), and remove the seeds. For masticating juicers, remove the peels and seeds; then chop to the size recommended by your juicer's instructions.
Jalapeño peppers	Rinse and remove the stems. Remove the seeds and white pith if you desire less heat.
Kale	Rinse thoroughly.
Kiwis	Scrub thoroughly or peel the outer layer.
Leaf lettuce	Rinse thoroughly and trim the base.
Lemons	If leaving the peel on, be sure to scrub the skin thoroughly. Otherwise, peel and quarter. The peel contains a lot of nutrients but can also impart bitterness to the juice.
Limes	If leaving the peel on, be sure to scrub the skin thoroughly. Otherwise, peel and quarter. The peel contains a lot of nutrients but can also impart some bitterness to the juice (though not as much as a lemon's).
Mangos	Peel and remove the pits.
Mint, all varieties	Rinse thoroughly and pat dry. Trim the ends of the stems and remove any blemished leaves.
Onions	Peel the papery outer layers.
Oranges	Peel and cut into a size appropriate to fit in your juicer.
Papayas	Peel and remove the seeds. ➤

➤ PRODUCE PREP CHART

Produce Variety	Preparation Instructions
Parsley	Rinse thoroughly and pat dry. Trim the ends of the stems and remove any blemished leaves.
Parsnips	Scrub and trim the tops.
Peaches	Wash and remove the pits.
Pears, all varieties	Rinse.
Pineapples	Scrub the outer layer. Remove the top and slice the full length of the fruit into 1-inch-thick stalks. If the core is extra woody or tough, remove it, but otherwise it is fine to include.
Plums	Rinse and remove the pits.
Pomegranates	Remove the outer husks and separate out the fleshy seeds.
Raspberries	Rinse.
Rhubarb	Remove the leaves as they are extremely poisonous. Rinse the stalks.
Romaine lettuce	Rinse thoroughly and trim the bottoms.
Scallions	Rinse and trim both ends.
Spinach	Wash extra thoroughly to remove grit.
Squash, summer	Wash and trim the woody stems.
Star fruit	Rinse.
Strawberries	Rinse thoroughly and remove any leaves that are dried out.
Sweet potatoes	Scrub thoroughly.

Produce Variety	Preparation Instructions
Swiss chard	Rinse.
Tomatoes	Rinse and remove any stems or leaves.
Turnips	Scrub and trim the tops.
Watercress	Rinse thoroughly.
Watermelon	Cut off the outer rind. Remove the largest seeds.
Wheatgrass	Rinse thoroughly and pat dry.

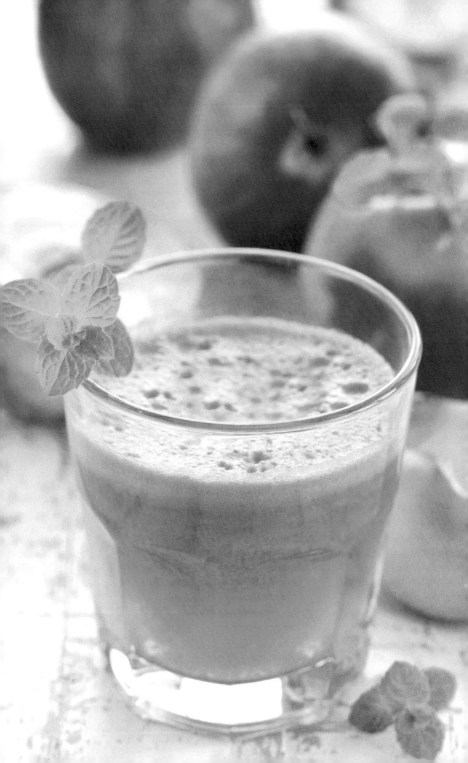

BREAKFAST JUICES

BREAKFAST MOJITO

NUTRITIONAL VALUES 50 CALORIES / 0G FAT / 1G PROTEIN

12G CARBS / 7G SUGAR / 10MG SODIUM

JUICER TYPE

This super-flavorful, super-low-calorie juice is like a nutrition-ist's dream cocktail. The cucumbers provide hydrating energy and antioxidants with a low dose of sugar. If you are sensitive to bitter flavors, you may wish to seed the cucumber and peel the lime, at least partially. However, these are some of the most antioxidant-rich parts of the fruit, so try to find a comfortable balance. If using a centrifugal juicer, double up on the basil or mint for about the same juice yield.

> 2 CUCUMBERS
> ½ CUP FIRMLY PACKED BASIL OR MINT LEAVES
> 1 LIME

Process all ingredients in your juicer and drink immediately for the best nutritional value. You can also store this juice in an airtight container in the refrigerator for up to 3 days.

Wake up the right way. All the juices in this chapter are designed to be a healthy and energizing way to kick off your day. Whether you want a healthy nutrition shot every morning or are trying to kick a coffee habit, the recipes here will help you start the day right.

SPINACH-CUCUMBER-CELERY

NUTRITIONAL VALUES   60 CALORIES / 1G FAT / 3G PROTEIN

9G CARBS / 3G SUGAR / 120MG SODIUM

JUICER TYPE

Give your morning a major nutritional kick-start with this hearty mixture. This juice features nutrient-dense spinach, complemented by the lighter and more aromatic cucumber and celery. All the ingredients in this juice have anti-inflammatory qualities, which are believed to provide a number of cardiovascular, joint, and other health benefits. This juice will give you an incredible start to the day and boasts a lower sugar content than most juices.

2 CUPS FIRMLY PACKED SPINACH
1 CUCUMBER
1 CELERY STALK

Process all ingredients in your juicer at once and drink immediately for the best nutritional value. You can also store this juice in an airtight container in the refrigerator for up to 1 day. While a centrifugal juicer is not recommended, you can get this recipe to work with one by adding the spinach first, and then slowly pushing the whole cucumber and celery down into the spinach as the juicer operates.

STRAWBERRY–ORANGE

NUTRITIONAL VALUES 110 CALORIES / 0G FAT / 1G PROTEIN

27G CARBS / 22G SUGAR / 2MG SODIUM

JUICER TYPE

You can't really go wrong nutrition-wise when it comes to berries, and strawberries are no exception. Packed with vitamin C and other antioxidants, these little superfood berries are a great way to start the day—and make for a very tasty juice. For an added health boost, toss in a small handful of spinach or kale (you won't even taste the difference).

> 2 ORANGES
> 1 CUP STRAWBERRIES

Process all ingredients in your juicer and drink immediately for the best nutritional value. You can also store this juice in an airtight container in the refrigerator for up to 3 days. For a thicker, more fiber-filled juice, juice the oranges separately (preferably in a citrus juicer), and then process the juice with fresh or frozen strawberries in a blender.

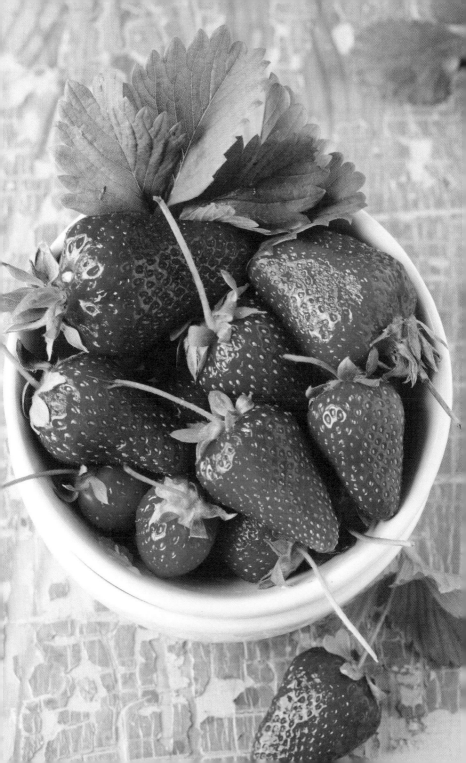

FRUITY VEGGIE JUICE

NUTRITIONAL VALUES 85 CALORIES / 1G FAT / 3G PROTEIN

17G CARBS / 11G SUGAR / 100MG SODIUM

JUICER TYPE

*This green vegetable juice is sweetened with fruit juices to make a
wonderfully energizing morning beverage. The parsley and ginger
add a healthy kick and a bit of bite. The cucumber is also a good
source of electrolytes, including potassium, to start your day off
hydrated (or at least compensate if you have a habit of drinking
too much coffee). If using a centrifugal juicer, sandwich the Swiss
chard or spinach between pieces of melon to extract as much juice
and nutrients as possible.*

1 CUCUMBER

1 CUP FIRMLY PACKED SWISS CHARD OR SPINACH

3 FLAT-LEAF PARSLEY SPRIGS

½ GRANNY SMITH APPLE

¾ CUP HONEYDEW MELON CUBES

1 CELERY STALK

¼ FENNEL BULB

1-INCH PIECE OF GINGER

Process all ingredients in your juicer and drink immediately
for the best nutritional value. You can also store this juice in
an airtight container in the refrigerator for up to 3 days.

GREEN ENERGY JUICE

NUTRITIONAL VALUES   90 CALORIES / 1G FAT / 5G PROTEIN

25G CARBS / 19G SUGAR / 45MG SODIUM

JUICER TYPE

The ingredients in this juice will give you an instant invigorating rush that won't fade. Kale is a great source of calcium and anti-oxidants, while apples provide electrolytes and the energy you need to get through the day. If you only have a centrifugal juicer, you can leave out the kale at first; then process it thoroughly with the juice in a blender to get the full nutrient dose and an added fiber bonus. You may never reach for coffee again.

5 LARGE KALE LEAVES
1 LEMON
2 APPLES
½-INCH PIECE OF GINGER
6 MINT LEAVES

Process all ingredients in your juicer and drink immediately for the best nutritional value. You can also store this juice in an airtight container in the refrigerator for up to 3 days.

ORANGE-CRANBERRY

NUTRITIONAL VALUES   100 CALORIES / 0G FAT / 1G PROTEIN

24G CARBS / 19G SUGAR / 3MG SODIUM

JUICER TYPE

Rather than added refined sugar, this juice uses naturally sweet oranges and apples to complement the very tart cranberries. Adding a little cucumber provides essential minerals while also making for a lighter, lower-calorie, and easier-to-drink breakfast juice.

  2 CUPS CRANBERRIES
  1 ORANGE
  1 APPLE
  1 CUCUMBER

Process all ingredients in your juicer and drink immediately for the best nutritional value. You can also store this juice in an airtight container in the refrigerator for up to 3 days.

PINEAPPLE–PAPAYA

NUTRITIONAL VALUES   170 CALORIES / OG FAT / 1G PROTEIN

42G CARBS / 30G SUGAR / 5MG SODIUM

JUICER TYPE

Feel free to vary the ratio of the two main fruits in this juice to suit your taste and convenience. Both fruits are high in enzymes that aid in the digestion of proteins, making this a great pairing with a heavy breakfast or if you regularly engage in intense exercise. Papaya also breaks down so thoroughly in a juicer that it thickens the juice to a nectar, making the beverage more filling.

    1 CUP CHOPPED PINEAPPLE
    1 CUP CHOPPED PAPAYA

Process all ingredients in your juicer and drink immediately for the best nutritional value. You can also store this juice in an airtight container in the refrigerator for up to 3 days.

A note on juicing papayas. *Papaya flesh nearly disintegrates in a juicer, lowering its yield and making for a thicker, richer-tasting juice. For any recipe involving papaya, you can also cut the papaya amount in half and put it in a blender with the juice of the remaining ingredients. A quick blitz of the blender will give you a rich, thick nectar full of fiber.*

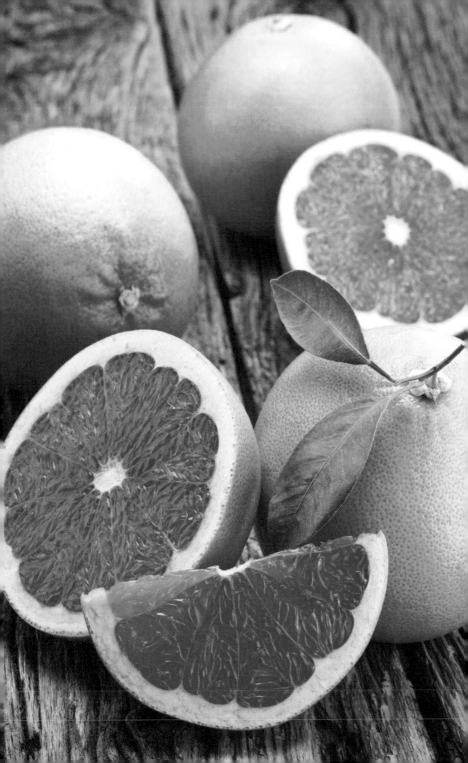

CITRUS WAKE-UP

NUTRITIONAL VALUES 160 CALORIES / 0G FAT / 2G PROTEIN

38G CARBS / 26G SUGAR / 80MG SODIUM

JUICER TYPE

This juice is a nutritionist's breakfast delight. It contains immense amounts of vitamins A and C, which are essential for fighting off infections. The carrots tone down the sugar rush of the citrus while providing soothing energy to wake you up gently. For best results, use a lower-acid, sweeter apple, such as Gala or Fuji.

1 GRAPEFRUIT
1 APPLE
3 OR 4 CARROTS
½-INCH PIECE OF GINGER
½ LEMON

Process all ingredients in your juicer and drink immediately for the best nutritional value. You can also store this juice in an airtight container in the refrigerator for up to 3 days.

ORANGE–BANANA

NUTRITIONAL VALUES 180 CALORIES / 1G FAT / 2G PROTEIN

42G CARBS / 32G SUGAR / 4MG SODIUM

JUICER TYPE

Bananas are high in fiber, potassium, and antioxidants. Oranges, high in vitamin C and potassium, are also a great way to bolster your immune system as you start the day. This smoothie-like juice will give you energy and keep you satisfied all morning. On hot days, try using a frozen banana (to freeze a banana, simply peel and put in a ziplock bag in the freezer for at least 4 hours).

> 2 ORANGES
> 1 RIPE BANANA, FRESH OR FROZEN

Process all ingredients in your juicer and drink immediately for the best nutritional value. Or juice the oranges (preferably in a citrus juicer) and then process the juice with the banana in a blender. You can store this juice in an airtight container in the refrigerator for up to 3 days.

GRAPEFRUIT, CARROT, AND GINGER

NUTRITIONAL VALUES   200 CALORIES / 1G FAT / 3G PROTEIN

42G CARBS / 23G SUGAR / 90MG SODIUM

JUICER TYPE

This juice provides a powerful energy shot full of antioxidants. The grapefruit is a good source of immune system–boosting vitamins A and C. Raw carrots retain far more nutritional value than cooked ones and provide a wide range of vitamins and fiber that will keep you full through the morning. And the ginger is a powerful anti-inflammatory agent that also aids digestion and can relieve symptoms of nausea.

1 LARGE GRAPEFRUIT
4 LARGE CARROTS
1–INCH PIECE OF GINGER

Process all ingredients in your juicer and drink immediately for the best nutritional value. You can also store this juice in an airtight container in the refrigerator for up to 3 days.

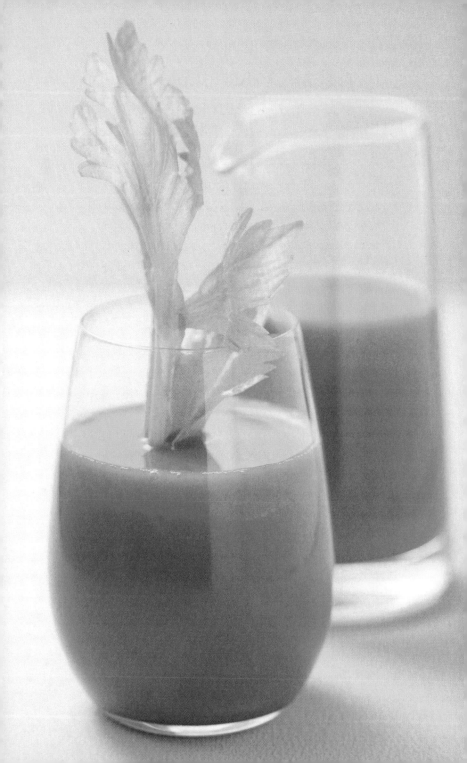

BRAIN-NOURISHING JUICES

CALMING VEGETABLE JUICE

NUTRITIONAL VALUES   60 CALORIES / 0G FAT / 3G PROTEIN

12G CARBS / 5G SUGAR / 25MG SODIUM

JUICER TYPE

This juice is packed with B and C vitamins that can help ease symptoms of depression and anxiety. Additionally, its infusion of essential minerals (such as calcium, iron, potassium, and zinc) may prevent anxiety and enhance feelings of calm. Finally, the complex carbohydrates in this juice give it a low glycemic index score, which helps maintain even blood sugar.

   2 TOMATOES
   ½ CUP FIRMLY PACKED PARSLEY
   1 RED BELL PEPPER
   2 CELERY STALKS
   3 BEET GREEN LEAVES OR ½ CUP FIRMLY PACKED
      SWISS CHARD

Process all ingredients in your juicer and drink immediately for the best nutritional value. You can also store this juice in an airtight container in the refrigerator for up to 3 days.

Body and mind.   Good nutrition is about both the body and the mind. This chapter focuses on juices that support mental health and brain function, whether that means relieving stress or headaches, improving cognitive ability, or diminishing symptoms of depression.

GREEN PICK-ME-UP

NUTRITIONAL VALUES 70 CALORIES / 1G FAT / 6G PROTEIN

8G CARBS / 2G SUGAR / 100MG SODIUM

JUICER TYPE

This very green, very healthful juice can be an acquired taste, but its amazing nutritional benefits make it well worth the effort. The ingredients provide a full day's supply of folic acid, and recent studies have shown that consuming healthy amounts of folic acid may reduce or even prevent many symptoms of depression. Even better, folic acid is also very important for a number of bodily and mental functions. Folic acid is especially important to consume while pregnant to help prevent certain birth defects.

2 CUPS CHOPPED BROCCOLI
½ CUP FIRMLY PACKED SPINACH
1 CUP SNOW PEAS
1 CUP FIRMLY PACKED SWISS CHARD
1 GREEN BELL PEPPER

Process all ingredients in your juicer and drink immediately for the best nutritional value. You can also store this juice in an airtight container in the refrigerator for up to 2 days.

CUCUMBER, CARROT, AND SPINACH

NUTRITIONAL VALUES 80 CALORIES / OG FAT / 4G PROTEIN

22G CARBS / 14G SUGAR / 80MG SODIUM

JUICER TYPE

Celery and cucumbers are both excellent sources of magnesium, which supports a healthy metabolism and acts as a natural muscle relaxant. The nutrients packed in this rich yet low-calorie juice have also been shown to help reduce migraine symptoms and possibly even prevent some migraines from occurring.

1 CUP FIRMLY PACKED SPINACH
1 CUCUMBER
3 CARROTS
2 CELERY STALKS (OPTIONAL)
PINCH OF SALT (OPTIONAL)

Process the first three ingredients in your juicer; if desired, add celery and stir in salt. Drink this juice immediately for the best nutritional value, or store in an airtight container in the refrigerator for up to 3 days.

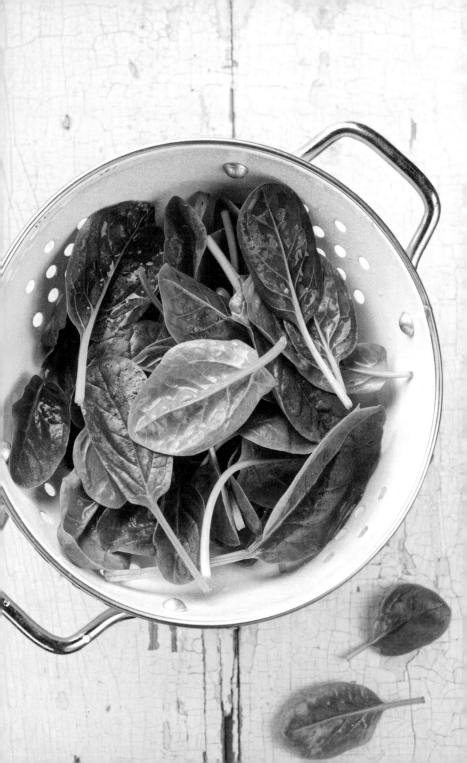

BRAIN HEALTH BOOST

NUTRITIONAL VALUES 130 CALORIES / 1G FAT / 3G PROTEIN

28G CARBS / 19G SUGAR / 80MG SODIUM

JUICER TYPE

All the ingredients in this juice have been shown to possibly help prevent or slow down the onset of Alzheimer's disease. If you have a centrifugal juicer and really want to make this juice, you can either double up on the spinach, or juice all the other ingredients first and then add ½ cup spinach and process the juice in a blender until smooth.

    1 CUP FIRMLY PACKED SPINACH
    1 CUP BLUEBERRIES
    1 CUP RASPBERRIES
    1 CUCUMBER
    1 TEASPOON TURMERIC (OPTIONAL)

Process the first four ingredients in your juicer and then stir in the turmeric, if desired. Drink immediately for the best nutritional value. You can also store this juice in an airtight container in the refrigerator for up to 3 days.

MORNING BRAIN BOOST

NUTRITIONAL VALUES   140 CALORIES / 1G FAT / 4G PROTEIN

30G CARBS / 15G SUGAR / 90MG SODIUM

JUICER TYPE

Beets, carrots, and spinach are all great sources of iron, zinc, and folic acid, all of which help the flow of oxygen to the brain. Maintaining healthy levels of these nutrients can improve brainpower, memory, and the ability to concentrate.

   3 CARROTS
   1 APPLE
   1 CUP FIRMLY PACKED SPINACH
   ½ RED BEET

Process all ingredients in your juicer and drink immediately for the best nutritional value. You can also store this juice in an airtight container in the refrigerator for up to 3 days.

STRESS AND HEADACHE RELIEF

NUTRITIONAL VALUES 140 CALORIES / 0G FAT / 3G PROTEIN

30G CARBS / 25G SUGAR / 40MG SODIUM

JUICER TYPE

Honeydew melons are a great source of iron, B vitamins, and many other essential nutrients. Melons in general have been shown to relieve stress and possibly even reduce headache symptoms. The high level of electrolytes and hydration this juice provides can also help prevent headaches and promote stress-free living.

    1½ CUPS CHOPPED HONEYDEW MELON
    1 ORANGE
    ½ CUP CHOPPED WATERMELON

Process all ingredients in your juicer and drink immediately for the best nutritional value. You can also store this juice in an airtight container in the refrigerator for up to 3 days.

WATERMELON–FENNEL

NUTRITIONAL VALUES   150 CALORIES / 1G FAT / 2G PROTEIN

33G CARBS / 27G SUGAR / 5MG SODIUM

JUICER TYPE

This juice can help in relieving stress, which will improve your focus and ability to sleep well. Fennel not only aids in digestion issues that can interfere with sleep, but also lowers stress. In addition to being packed with vitamin C, watermelon has been shown to relieve sore muscles and other mild aches and pains.

2 CUPS CHOPPED WATERMELON
2 OR 3 ROMAINE LETTUCE LEAVES
½ FENNEL BULB

Process all ingredients in your juicer and drink immediately for the best nutritional value. You can also store this juice in an airtight container in the refrigerator for up to 3 days.

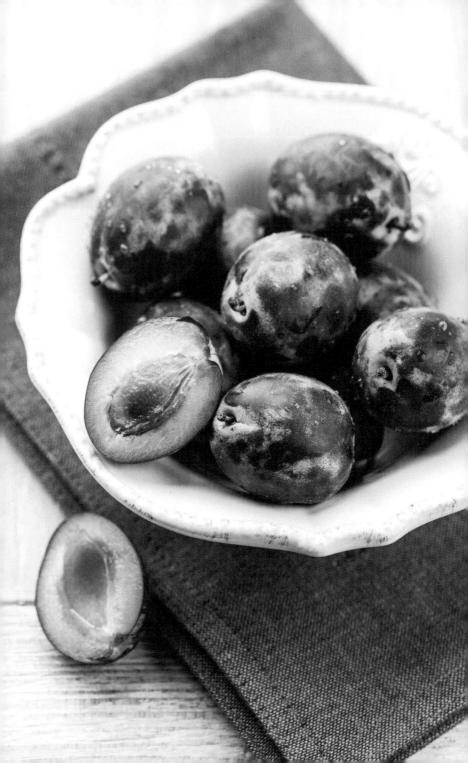

CALMING CHERRY–PLUM

NUTRITIONAL VALUES   160 CALORIES / 1G FAT / 1G PROTEIN

35G CARBS / 25G SUGAR / 10MG SODIUM

JUICER TYPE

Tart cherries are somewhat new on the superfoods block, but they have certainly made a big splash. Tart cherries are very high in melatonin, a compound that helps slow aging, improves sleep, and can relieve jet lag. Additional studies are underway exploring its role in reducing the risk of cancer and depression. The many health benefits of this delicious juice make it well worth the extra prepping required.

    1 CUP TART CHERRIES, PITTED
    3 LARGE DARK PLUMS
    1 APPLE
    ½ CUP FIRMLY PACKED SPINACH (OPTIONAL)

Process all ingredients in your juicer and drink immediately for the best nutritional value. You can also store this juice in an airtight container in the refrigerator for up to 3 days.

How to pit cherries without a cherry pitter. One simple way to pit a cherry without a proper cherry pitter is to get a metal funnel and place it upside down on the counter. Then place a stemmed cherry on the funnel tube (stemmed end down) and push down.

MANGO–CARROT FOCUS

NUTRITIONAL VALUES 170 CALORIES / 0G FAT / 4G PROTEIN

40G CARBS / 33G SUGAR / 100MG SODIUM

JUICER TYPE

Carrots are an incredibly good source of vitamin A, particularly in its beta-carotene form, which is a powerful antioxidant that may combat the brain's aging process and improve focus. This juice is also a good source of selenium, which helps with concentration and maintaining a proper metabolism.

1 MANGO, CHOPPED

3 CARROTS

½ APPLE

Process all ingredients in your juicer and drink immediately for the best nutritional value. You can also store this juice in an airtight container in the refrigerator for up to 3 days.

Mango caution. *Mangos are loosely related to poison ivy and excrete a similar compound in the skin of their fruits. While generally harmless (though not pleasant tasting), it can cause a painful rash in people who are especially sensitive to it. Always peel mangos completely before juicing.*

TOMATO–APPLE
ALERT JUICE

NUTRITIONAL VALUES 280 CALORIES / 19G FAT / 8G PROTEIN

18G CARBS / 11G SUGAR / 2MG SODIUM

JUICER TYPE

Did you know that your brain needs a steady supply of natural fats in order to operate at top efficiency? Walnuts and flaxseed are two of the best sources of heart- and brain-healthy fats. Additionally, this juice is high in B vitamins and folate, which are important for maintaining brain health. If you are concerned about calories, it is fine to reduce the walnuts and flaxseed oil by half.

  1 APPLE
  1 TOMATO
  1 CUP WATER
  3 TABLESPOONS CHOPPED WALNUTS
  1 TEASPOON FLAXSEED OIL

Juice the apple and tomato; then transfer the juice to a blender. Add the water, walnuts, and flaxseed oil and process until smooth. Drink immediately for the best nutritional value, or store this juice in an airtight container in the refrigerator for up to 3 days.

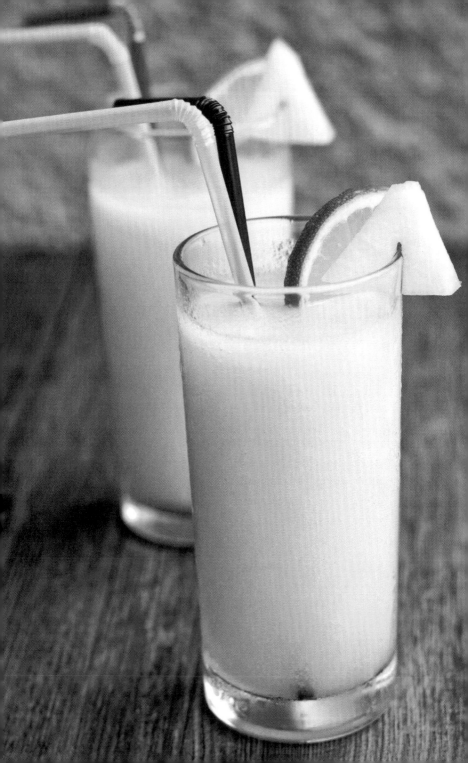

5

ALKALIZING
JUICES

SIMPLE ALKALIZER

NUTRITIONAL VALUES   50 CALORIES / 0G FAT / 1G PROTEIN

12G CARBS / 7G SUGAR / 3MG SODIUM

JUICER TYPE

In this refresher, the highly alkalizing properties of cucumber and celery are combined with the slightly alkalizing lemon. It's a bright, fresh juice that is especially enjoyable over ice on a hot summer's day. Although acidic themselves, lemons actually act to help alkalize the body. Be sure to include the peel when juicing to get all the nutrients and benefits.

    1 CUCUMBER
    1 LEMON
    4 CELERY STALKS

Process all ingredients in your juicer and drink immediately for the best nutritional value. You can also store this juice in an airtight container in the refrigerator for up to 3 days.

SPINACH-FENNEL

NUTRITIONAL VALUES   60 CALORIES / 0G FAT / 4G PROTEIN

11G CARBS / 6G SUGAR / 350MG SODIUM

JUICER TYPE

Spinach is one of the most alkalizing foods you will find, but it can also be hard to juice. Fennel and cucumber provide electrolytes and hydration while serving as a great base for the spinach (and are also alkalizing on their own). Sandwiching the spinach between thick slices of fennel and cucumber can make this juice worth a try even with a centrifugal juicer, but you may want to add another cup of spinach to increase the yield.

2 CUPS FIRMLY PACKED SPINACH
1 GARLIC CLOVE
1 FENNEL BULB
1 CUCUMBER
½ LEMON

Process all ingredients in your juicer and drink immediately for the best nutritional value. You can also store this juice in an airtight container in the refrigerator for up to 3 days.

Alkalizing tips. Almost all green vegetables are great for people on alkalizing diets. See Chapter 12, "Green Juices," for many more delicious and nutritious juices that will complement your diet.

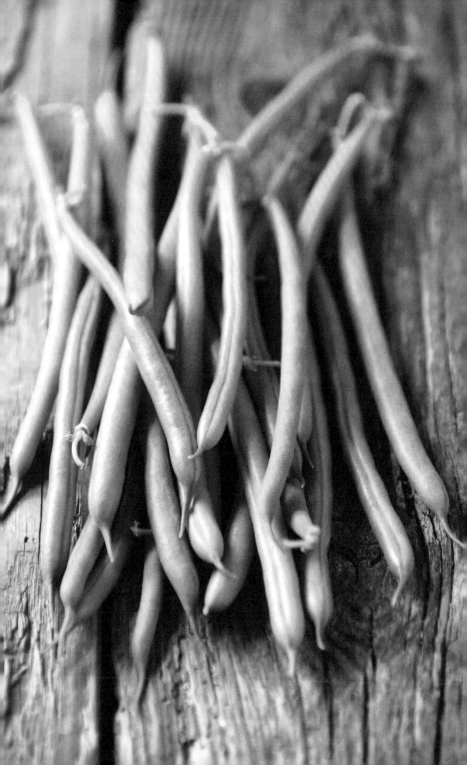

SPRING HARVEST ALKALIZER

NUTRITIONAL VALUES 60 CALORIES / 0G FAT / 2G PROTEIN

13G CARBS / 4G SUGAR / 20MG SODIUM

JUICER TYPE

If you like to garden, this is a great juice to make with early harvest vegetables. For an added boost, you can throw in some spring greens as well. In addition, when basil is allowed to grow a bit wild, it will often begin to flower. These flower buds and seeds are too tough to use as an herb in cooking, but work really well in a juicer!

1 CUP YELLOW OR GREEN BEANS
1 CUP SNOW PEAS
1 GARLIC CLOVE
1 SCALLION
½ CUP ALFALFA SPROUTS
¼ CUP FIRMLY PACKED BASIL
½ LEMON

Process all ingredients in your juicer and drink immediately for the best nutritional value. You can also store this juice in an airtight container in the refrigerator for up to 3 days.

SPICY ALKALIZING
TOMATO JUICE

NUTRITIONAL VALUES   70 CALORIES / OG FAT / 1G PROTEIN

17G CARBS / 5G SUGAR / 2MG SODIUM

JUICER TYPE

Even if you don't care about alkalizing, this is a fantastic juice that
even makes a great mixer for a Bloody Mary if you toss in some
horseradish! Look for a chile that is red and ripe for the best flavor
and antioxidant boost.

1 LEMON
1 JALAPEÑO PEPPER OR OTHER CHILE
1 CELERY STALK
2 TOMATOES
1 CUCUMBER
½ CUP PEAS

Process all ingredients in your juicer and drink immediately
for the best nutritional value. You can also store this juice in
an airtight container in the refrigerator for up to 3 days.

SUMMER HARVEST ALKALIZER

NUTRITIONAL VALUES   75 CALORIES / 1G FAT / 6G PROTEIN

14G CARBS / 3G SUGAR / 70MG SODIUM

JUICER TYPE

Most fresh green herbs provide alkalizing benefits. This juice makes use of common summer harvest vegetables that often overflow the garden. When trimming broccoli, be sure to to save the juice-rich stems—while not as nutrient-dense as the florets, broccoli stems are still a great protein and electrolyte source.

> 1½ CUPS CHOPPED BROCCOLI
> 1 TOMATO
> 1 BELL PEPPER (ANY COLOR)
> 2 CARROTS
> 1 CELERY STALK
> ½ CUP FIRMLY PACKED PARSLEY
> PINCH OF SALT (OPTIONAL)

Process the first six ingredients in your juicer; then stir in the salt if desired. Drink this juice immediately for the best nutritional value, or store in an airtight container in the refrigerator for up to 2 days.

POWER ALKALIZER

NUTRITIONAL VALUES   190 CALORIES / 1G FAT / 7G PROTEIN

35G CARBS / 15G SUGAR / 110MG SODIUM

JUICER TYPE

This juice pays less attention to flavor and more to being an aggressively powerful alkalizer. If you have strayed from the healthful path and need a power shot to get you back on track, give this juice a try. Because cabbage juice spoils quickly, it's best to drink this juice freshly made.

2 CELERY STALKS
1 CUP FIRMLY PACKED SPINACH
½ HEAD GREEN CABBAGE
1 BELL PEPPER (ANY COLOR)
½ CUP FIRMLY PACKED WHEATGRASS

Process all ingredients in your juicer and drink immediately for the best nutritional value. You can also store this juice in an airtight container in the refrigerator for up to 1 day, but it is not recommended.

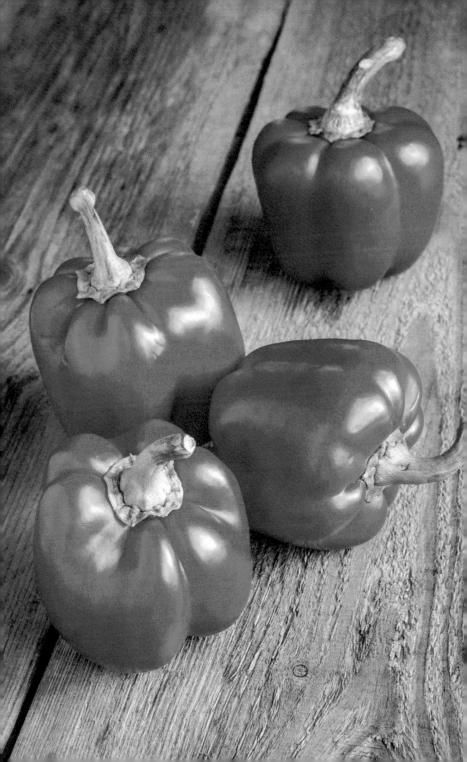

SWEET VEGETABLE JUICE

NUTRITIONAL VALUES 105 CALORIES / 0G FAT / 1G PROTEIN

26G CARBS / 13G SUGAR / 160MG SODIUM

JUICER TYPE

To adhere to a diet with at least 80 percent of your food in the alkalizing category, you generally need to avoid sugars. The vegetables in this juice provide strong alkalizing properties while still offering a sweet-tasting treat. Salad turnips have a similar flavor to radishes but are much milder. Both radish and turnip greens are also incredibly nourishing—just be sure they are fresh, with no rotten or brown spots.

4 CARROTS
8 SALAD TURNIPS OR RADISHES, INCLUDING GREENS
1 RED BEET

Process all ingredients in your juicer and drink immediately for the best nutritional value. You can also store this juice in an airtight container in the refrigerator for up to 3 days.

ALKALIZING FRUIT JUICE

NUTRITIONAL VALUES   120 CALORIES / 0G FAT / 0G PROTEIN

30G CARBS / 20G SUGAR / 5MG SODIUM

JUICER TYPE

Though all these fruits are technically acidic themselves, once in the body they aid in alkalization. This refreshing and fruity juice is a great alternative to the many vegetal and earthy green juices you'll typically find in an alkalizing diet. While this juice won't provide as strong an alkalizing punch, it will keep you going in the right direction.

> 1 GRAPEFRUIT
> ½ LEMON
> 1 CUP CHOPPED WATERMELON

Process all ingredients in your juicer and drink immediately for the best nutritional value. You can also store this juice in an airtight container in the refrigerator for up to 3 days.

Enhance your alkaline juice even further. Chia sprouts, almonds, and avocados are all great alkaline ingredients that go well in many juices. These ingredients do not juice well; it is best to process these ingredients in a blender first, and then combine with prepared juice.

ALKALIZING VEGGIE JUICE

NUTRITIONAL VALUES 140 CALORIES / 2G FAT / 11G PROTEIN

24G CARBS / 8G SUGAR / 130MG SODIUM

JUICER TYPE

A challenge with alkaline juices is to combine the alkaline ingredients in a way that is enjoyable to drink. Broccoli is incredibly nutritious and alkalizing, but not the most enjoyable juice to consume on its own. In this recipe, carrots add sweetness, cucumber and celery lighten the bold flavor considerably, and together with the broccoli, produce a juice with powerful alkalizing properties.

3 CUPS CHOPPED BROCCOLI

3 CARROTS

2 CELERY STALKS

½ CUCUMBER

PINCH OF SALT (OPTIONAL)

Process the first four ingredients in your juicer; then stir in the salt if desired. Drink this juice immediately for the best nutritional value, or store in an airtight container in the refrigerator for up to 2 days.

GREEN BALANCE

NUTRITIONAL VALUES   140 CALORIES / 2G FAT / 4G PROTEIN

30G CARBS / 15G SUGAR / 105MG SODIUM

JUICER TYPE

*This juice is pleasant and light, despite not being very sweet
at all. Its ingredients are all alkaline, while its low sugar load
makes it low on the glycemic index as well. To make this juice
using a centrifugal juicer, process everything but the basil. In a
blender, combine only the most tender basil leaves with the juice,
pulsing until smooth.*

> 5 TO 7 KALE LEAVES
> 1 CUCUMBER
> 1 FENNEL BULB
> 3 CARROTS
> ½-INCH PIECE OF GINGER
> ½ CUP FIRMLY PACKED BASIL

Process all ingredients in your juicer and drink immediately
for the best nutritional value. You can also store this juice in
an airtight container in the refrigerator for up to 3 days.

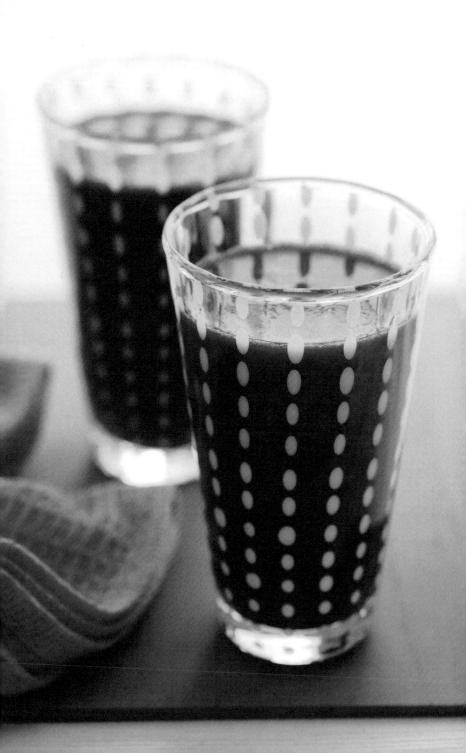

ANTI-AGING JUICES

TOMATO TONIC

NUTRITIONAL VALUES 65 CALORIES / 1G FAT / 2G PROTEIN

14G CARBS / 7G SUGAR / 60MG SODIUM

JUICER TYPE

Recent studies have shown that tomatoes protect the skin against sun damage and even help the skin heal faster from sun damage. This ultimately results in skin that defies aging. The antioxidants found in this juice also help neutralize free radicals in the body, which contribute to aging and other health problems.

2 TOMATOES
1 CUCUMBER
½-INCH PIECE OF GINGER
1 GARLIC CLOVE (OPTIONAL)

Process all ingredients in your juicer and drink immediately for the best nutritional value. You can also store this juice in an airtight container in the refrigerator for up to 3 days.

Top anti-aging foods. Any diet rich in fresh, antioxidant-rich fruits and vegetables will help you maintain a youthful look and energy level. However, studies have shown that dark-skinned berries, beans and bean sprouts, leafy greens, avocados, nuts, and garlic contain compounds and nutrients that are particularly good at helping you stay vibrant and active.

SPROUTS FOR HAIR HEALTH

NUTRITIONAL VALUES 80 CALORIES / 1G FAT / OG PROTEIN

18G CARBS / 13G SUGAR / 2MG SODIUM

JUICER TYPE

The sprouts in this recipe include minerals and other nutrients essential for healthy, shiny hair and nails. Feel free to mix, match, and substitute the various sprouts for similar benefits, but the alfalfa sprouts should be prioritized for best results. Because the sprouts are so small and light, a centrifugal juicer is not recommended for this recipe. For additional anti-aging benefits and fewer calories, replace the grapes with 2 carrots.

 1 CUCUMBER
 1 CUP RED GRAPES
 1 CUP ALFALFA SPROUTS
 ½ CUP RADISH SPROUTS
 ½ CUP BEAN SPROUTS
 ½ CUP CLOVER SPROUTS

Process all ingredients in your juicer and drink immediately for the best nutritional value. You can also store this juice in an airtight container in the refrigerator for up to 3 days.

BEET THE CLOCK

NUTRITIONAL VALUES 105 CALORIES / 0G FAT / 2G PROTEIN

25G CARBS / 17G SUGAR / 80MG SODIUM

JUICER TYPE

*Beets are rich in vitamins and minerals, including vitamins
A and C, fiber, folate, manganese, and potassium. Foods high
in folate have been shown to help prevent and minimize wrinkles. This juice is filled with antioxidants, which revive your
body's cells while supporting liver and brain function. Ginger
and lemons are also very high in vitamin C and have strong
anti-inflammatory properties, which help promote smooth,
wrinkle-free skin.*

    1 OR 2 RED BEETS
    1 HEAD LEAF LETTUCE
    1 APPLE
    1 LEMON
    ½-INCH PIECE OF GINGER

Process all ingredients in your juicer and drink immediately
for the best nutritional value. You can also store this juice in
an airtight container in the refrigerator for up to 3 days.

TURNIP, FENNEL, AND PARSNIP YOUTHFUL TONIC

NUTRITIONAL VALUES   120 CALORIES / 1G FAT / 4G PROTEIN

24G CARBS / 14G SUGAR / 80MG SODIUM

JUICER TYPE

Don't let the ingredient list scare you! Parsnips are actually sweeter than carrots, and a great source of folate, vitamin C, and manganese, which collectively help promote skin and eye health and soothe the nervous system. The recipe is also tempered with apples to ease the strong taste of turnip. The turnip and fennel aid in cleansing the liver, help prevent kidney stones, and may even reduce the risk of certain cancers. Fennel aids digestion and helps treat anemia.

1½ CUPS CHOPPED TURNIP
3 PARSNIPS
1 APPLE
½ FENNEL BULB

Process all ingredients in your juicer and drink immediately for the best nutritional value. You can also store this juice in an airtight container in the refrigerator for up to 3 days.

GREEN FOUNTAIN OF YOUTH

NUTRITIONAL VALUES 200 CALORIES / 3G FAT / 1G PROTEIN

45G CARBS / 28G SUGAR / 10MG SODIUM

JUICER TYPE

Cabbage is one of the healthiest vegetables you will find. This superstar of superfoods provides a wealth of anti-aging benefits. Both green and purple vegetables include important compounds that help improve complexions and fight the aging process. The surprisingly light-tasting and sweet purple cabbage in this juice helps promote cardiovascular and brain health while providing an ample supply of anti-aging antioxidants.

2 CUPS CHOPPED PURPLE CABBAGE

1 CUP FIRMLY PACKED SPINACH

2 CELERY STALKS

½ BUNCH KALE

1 LEMON

2 APPLES

½-INCH PIECE OF GINGER

Process all ingredients in your juicer and drink immediately for the best nutritional value. You can also store this juice in an airtight container in the refrigerator for up to 2 days.

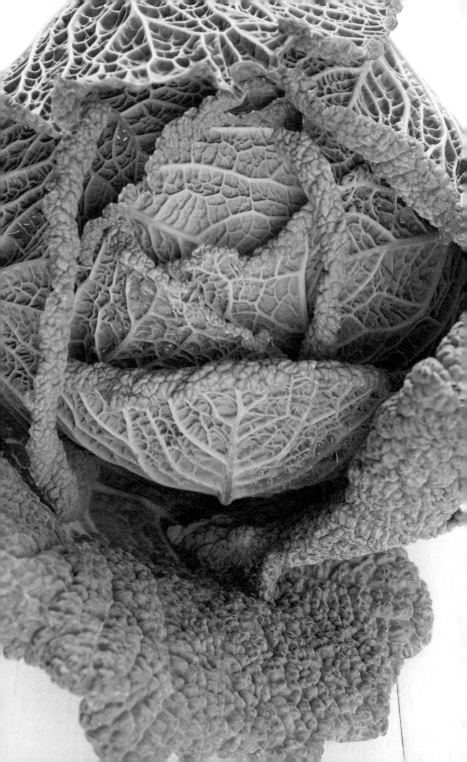

SUPERFOOD SUPERJUICE

NUTRITIONAL VALUES   130 CALORIES / 1G FAT / 7G PROTEIN

29G CARBS / 20G SUGAR / 10MG SODIUM

JUICER TYPE   C M T

This juice combines dark leafy greens with dark-skinned berries. These superfoods contain high levels of antioxidants to neutralize free radicals, which are thought to contribute to the aging process. This juice also includes ingredients that promote healthy skin, hair, and nails, while providing a mood-boosting energy enhancement.

    1 CUP BLACKBERRIES
    1 CUP STRAWBERRIES
    ½ CUP BLUEBERRIES
    ½ CUP RASPBERRIES
    1 CUP CHOPPED PINEAPPLE
    1 CUP FIRMLY PACKED SPINACH

Process all ingredients in your juicer and drink immediately for the best nutritional value. You can also store this juice in an airtight container in the refrigerator for up to 3 days.

REJUVENATING MORNING

NUTRITIONAL VALUES 130 CALORIES / 2G FAT / 1G PROTEIN

34G CARBS / 15G SUGAR / 80MG SODIUM

JUICER TYPE

*All the ingredients in this delicious juice contribute to healthy
skin and eyes and improve the metabolism, making this beverage
a great way to start every day! The high level of antioxidants
found in the carrots and kale help tighten skin, while the ginger
helps reduce inflammation. Coconut milk is high in skin-healthy
vitamin E, healthy fats, essential minerals, and anti-inflammatory
properties that will help you feel and look healthy.*

2 CARROTS
1 APPLE
2 KALE LEAVES
¼-INCH PIECE OF GINGER
¼ CUP COCONUT MILK

Process the first four ingredients in your juicer and then combine with the coconut milk, stirring or shaking well to blend.
Drink immediately for the best nutritional value, or store in
an airtight container in the refrigerator for up to 3 days.

Making your own coconut milk is quick and easy!
Simply combine about 2 cups dried, unsweetened coconut shreds
with 2 cups water in a saucepan and simmer for about 10 minutes.
Pour through a cheesecloth or nut milk bag to separate out all
the fiber. This coconut milk will remain fresh for about 3 days
when refrigerated.

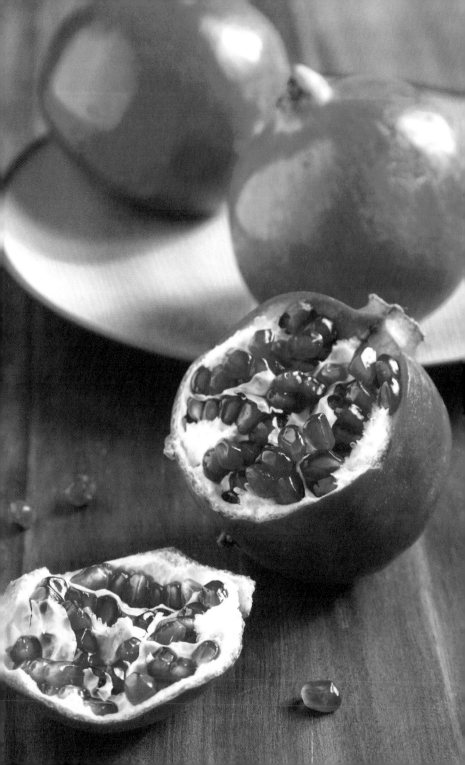

ANTIOXIDANT POWER JUICE

NUTRITIONAL VALUES   145 CALORIES / 0G FAT / 0G PROTEIN

36G CARBS / 30G SUGAR / 8MG SODIUM

JUICER TYPE

The blueberries and pomegranates in this juice are superfoods containing incredibly high levels of antioxidants. These antioxidants are thought to neutralize free radicals in the body that contribute to aging skin and organs. The vitamin C found in all the ingredients helps form and maintain collagen, contributing to firm skin and muscles.

JUICY SEEDS OF 1 POMEGRANATE
1 CUP BLUEBERRIES
1 CUP STRAWBERRIES
1 APPLE

Process all ingredients in your juicer and drink immediately for the best nutritional value. You can also store this juice in an airtight container in the refrigerator for up to 3 days.

MENOPAUSE RELIEF AND SUPPORT

NUTRITIONAL VALUES 160 CALORIES / 0G FAT / 1G PROTEIN

39G CARBS / 30G SUGAR / 5MG SODIUM

JUICER TYPE

A common recommendation for any woman seeking to ease meno-pause symptoms is simply to eat more fruits and veggies, which any juice in this book will help with. However, the ingredients in this juice are all great sources of boron, which helps counteract estrogen loss while reducing risk of osteoporosis.

1 CUP RED GRAPES
2 PEARS (PREFERABLY ANJOU OR RED)
1 CUP STRAWBERRIES

Process all ingredients in your juicer and drink immediately for the best nutritional value. You can also store this juice in an airtight container in the refrigerator for up to 3 days.

BACK TO SPRING GREENS

NUTRITIONAL VALUES 180 CALORIES / 1G FAT / 1G PROTEIN

30G CARBS / 20G SUGAR / 20MG SODIUM

JUICER TYPE

This packs as powerful an antioxidant punch as any green juice does, but with a lighter and brighter taste. Parsley has amazing cleansing properties that can help improve digestive health. The nutrients in this juice also help reduce wrinkles, increase mental alertness, and revitalize the metabolism. If you enjoy the ginger's flavor, feel free to double the quantity to take advantage of its anti-inflammatory properties.

1 PEAR

1 APPLE

1 CUP FIRMLY PACKED SPINACH

½ CUP FIRMLY PACKED PARSLEY

½ CUCUMBER

1 CELERY STALK

½-INCH PIECE OF GINGER

Process all ingredients in your juicer and drink immediately for the best nutritional value. You can also store this juice in an airtight container in the refrigerator for up to 3 days.

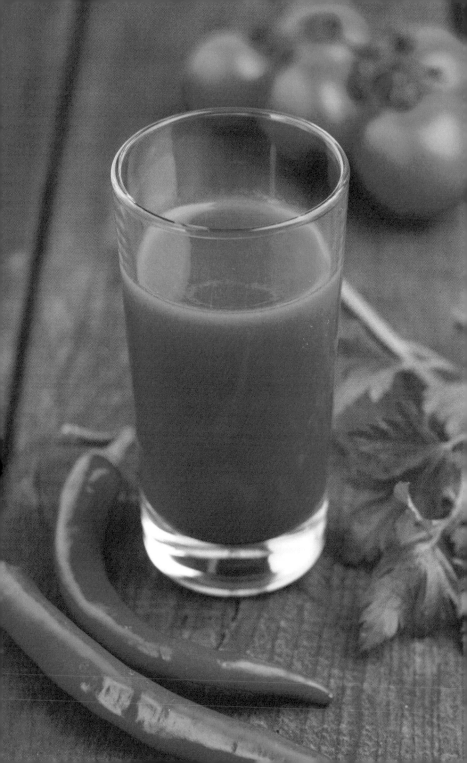

7

ANTIOXIDANT JUICES

GARLIC INFUSION

NUTRITIONAL VALUES 50 CALORIES / 0G FAT / 1G PROTEIN

12G CARBS / 4G SUGAR / 20MG SODIUM

JUICER TYPE

The health and medicinal benefits of garlic have been known for centuries. Raw garlic works as a natural antibiotic that can fight off many strains of harmful bacteria. Garlic can also decrease blood pressure, remove heavy metals from the body, and possibly even prevent certain cancers. Every clove of garlic contains high levels of vitamins A, B, and C; iron; calcium; iodine; potassium; selenium; zinc; and magnesium. Tomatoes and cucumbers are also great sources of vitamin C and other antioxidants, including cancer-fighting lycopene.

    3 GARLIC CLOVES
    3 TOMATOES
    1 CUCUMBER
    ¼ CUP FIRMLY PACKED PARSLEY
    PINCH OF SALT (OPTIONAL)

Process the first four ingredients in your juicer; then stir in the salt if desired. Drink this juice immediately for the best nutritional value, or store in an airtight container in the refrigerator for up to 3 days.

What is an antioxidant? *An antioxidant is a molecule that inhibits the oxidation of other molecules. In the human body, oxidation can produce free radicals, which are rogue molecules that can damage healthy cells. Free radicals can cause everything from premature aging to cancer. A diet packed with antioxidants helps neutralize these free radicals.*

SPICY TOMATO

NUTRITIONAL VALUES 60 CALORIES / 1G FAT / 1G PROTEIN

14G CARBS / 5G SUGAR / 80MG SODIUM

JUICER TYPE

Many varieties of peppers contain up to ten times the vitamin C antioxidant punch of an orange! Tomatoes are by far the best food source of lycopene, an antioxidant being touted as possibly even a more powerful disease fighter than vitamin E or beta-carotene. This juice is a delicious low-calorie source of antioxidants.

    1 JALAPEÑO PEPPER OR OTHER CHILE
    4 OR 5 TOMATOES
    ¼ RED ONION
    1 GARLIC CLOVE
    PINCH OF SALT (OPTIONAL)

Process the first four ingredients in your juicer; then stir in the salt if desired. Drink this juice immediately for the best nutritional value, or store in an airtight container in the refrigerator for up to 3 days.

Unlocking the health benefits of tomatoes. *The human body needs fats in order to properly absorb and utilize lycopene, so it is recommended that you pair your tomato juice antioxidant supply with a meal that provides a good source of unsaturated fats, such as salmon or beans. Another option is to stir a teaspoon of flaxseed oil into the juice.*

STRAWBERRY, PAPAYA, AND ORANGE

NUTRITIONAL VALUES   90 CALORIES / 0G FAT / 2G PROTEIN

28G CARBS / 17G SUGAR / 3MG SODIUM

JUICER TYPE

It would be hard to top this juice when looking for a good source of vitamin C, both in nutritional quality and flavor! Be certain to peel the papaya before juicing; its peel contains compounds that can upset your stomach and add excessively bitter flavors to the juice.

1 CUP CHOPPED PAPAYA
1 ORANGE
1 CUP STRAWBERRIES

Process all ingredients in your juicer and drink immediately for the best nutritional value. You can also store this juice in an airtight container in the refrigerator for up to 3 days.

VEGETABLE VITAMIN KICK

NUTRITIONAL VALUES 90 CALORIES / 1G FAT / 7G PROTEIN

18G CARBS / 9G SUGAR / 70MG SODIUM

JUICER TYPE

Lycopene is an antioxidant that may help reduce the risk of several types of cancer, including prostate, ovarian, and cervical. Bright red and ripe tomatoes are a great source. Fruits and vegetables that are high in color are generally high in nutrition and packed with antioxidants. When selecting produce, aim to include a mix of greens, reds, oranges, and other bright colors to get nutritional variety and maximum health benefits.

2 TOMATOES
1 CELERY STALK
1 RED BEET
½ CUP FIRMLY PACKED PARSLEY
2 GARLIC CLOVES
1 CARROT
½ LEMON
2 ASPARAGUS SPEARS (OPTIONAL)

Process all ingredients in your juicer and drink immediately for the best nutritional value. You can also store this juice in an airtight container in the refrigerator for up to 3 days.

ROOTS AND SHOOTS

NUTRITIONAL VALUES 90 CALORIES / 1G FAT / 4G PROTEIN

16G CARBS / 7G SUGAR / 40MG SODIUM

JUICER TYPE

Asparagus is a great source of nutrients, including folate, vitamin A, and vitamin K. This spring shoot also packs a healthy protein punch. This tasty juice provides a great source of vitamins A, B, C, and E as well as other antioxidants. Feel free to garnish with salt, pepper, and a wedge of lime.

3 ASPARAGUS SPEARS
1 RED BEET
2 CARROTS
1 TOMATO
1 CELERY STALK

Process all ingredients in your juicer and drink immediately for the best nutritional value. You can also store this juice in an airtight container in the refrigerator for up to 3 days.

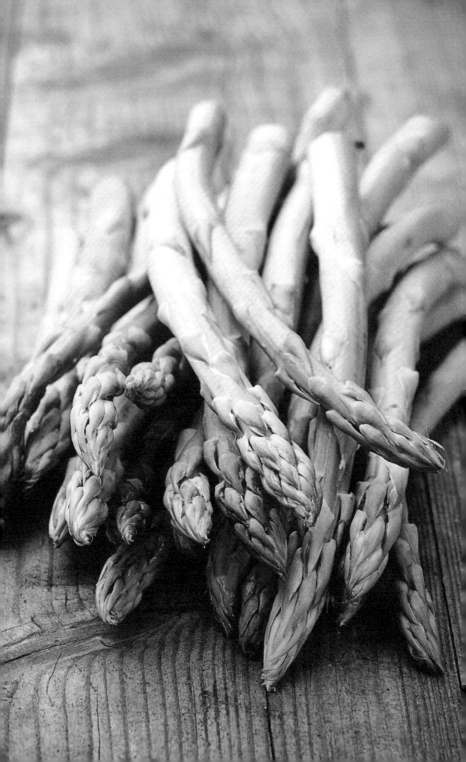

KIWI–PEAR–STRAWBERRY

NUTRITIONAL VALUES 110 CALORIES / 0G FAT / 1G PROTEIN

27G CARBS / 19G SUGAR / 1MG SODIUM

JUICER TYPE

Just one kiwi contains more than 100 percent of the recommended daily intake of vitamin C, a powerful antioxidant. This juice, which makes a refreshing summer treat, is also packed with a number of B vitamins. The skin of the kiwi is the most antioxidant rich part of the fruit, but will also make the juice quite sour. To test your limits, try adding the kiwis to your juicer one by one, sampling the juice after each addition.

3 KIWIS
1 PEAR
1 CUP STRAWBERRIES
½ LEMON

Process all ingredients in your juicer and drink immediately for the best nutritional value. You can also store this juice in an airtight container in the refrigerator for up to 3 days.

PEACHY GRAPE

NUTRITIONAL VALUES 140 CALORIES / 1G FAT / 3G PROTEIN

32G CARBS / 28G SUGAR / 5MG SODIUM

JUICER TYPE

Grapes are a great source of vitamins B, C, and K, and of course, are sweet and delicious. Peaches are a good source of antioxidants and potassium, and when juiced, break down into a sweet nectar. Be sure to remove the pits from peaches and other stone fruits before putting them in your juicer—otherwise you might need to buy a new one!

    2 CUPS GREEN GRAPES
    2 PEACHES
    ½ LEMON

Process all ingredients in your juicer and drink immediately for the best nutritional value. You can also store this juice in an airtight container in the refrigerator for up to 3 days.

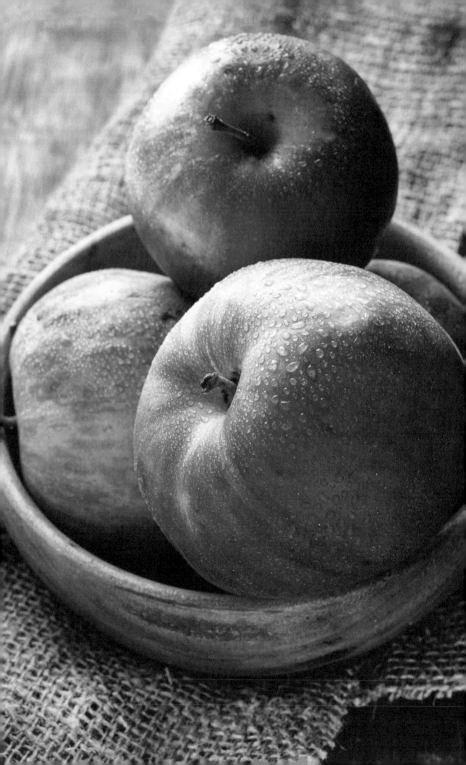

BROCCOLI, APPLE, AND BERRY

NUTRITIONAL VALUES 140 CALORIES / 1G FAT / 7G PROTEIN

26G CARBS / 18G SUGAR / 60MG SODIUM

JUICER TYPE

Broccoli is a great source of vitamins A, B, and C and is considered one of the world's healthiest foods for its nutritional density. Broccoli also contains a compound called sulforaphane, which boosts enzymes thought to protect the body from cancer-causing chemicals. In addition, the berries and fruit in this juice contain superfood levels of antioxidants. Although the lemon peel contains a very bitter pith, it is a valuable source of bioflavonoids and other nutrients.

> 1 CUP CHOPPED BROCCOLI
> 2 APPLES
> ½ CUP CRANBERRIES
> ½ CUP STRAWBERRIES
> ½ LEMON

Process all ingredients in your juicer and drink immediately for the best nutritional value. You can also store this juice in an airtight container in the refrigerator for up to 2 days.

SUPERFOOD BERRY BLAST

NUTRITIONAL VALUES 140 CALORIES / 1G FAT / 4G PROTEIN

34G CARBS / 30G SUGAR / 5MG SODIUM

JUICER TYPE

Dark-skinned berries are widely considered one of the best sources of antioxidants, particularly vitamin C. Blueberries are considered a superfood; they are a great source of flavonoids, compounds currently being studied with great interest due to their antioxidant properties. They are thought to neutralize free radicals, preventing coronary heart disease and reduce the risk of cancer.

    1 CUP BLACKBERRIES
    1 CUP BLUEBERRIES
    1 CUP DARK-SKINNED GRAPES
    1 APPLE

Process all ingredients in your juicer and drink immediately for the best nutritional value. You can also store this juice in an airtight container in the refrigerator for up to 3 days.

Best antioxidant sources. Virtually all fresh fruits and vegetables contain antioxidants, some more so than others. Berries, broccoli, garlic, tomatoes, and leafy greens are especially powerful sources. Because many antioxidants break down when exposed to heat, juicing is the perfect way to capture these nutrients in abundance.

CITRUS VITAMIN C

NUTRITIONAL VALUES 180 CALORIES / OG FAT / 1G PROTEIN

44G CARBS / 37G SUGAR / 5MG SODIUM

JUICER TYPE

The very sweet and tart flavors of the citrus in this juice allow you to spike it with vitamin D-rich spinach—with no appreciable difference in taste. A nutrient-dense superfood, spinach certainly boosts the antioxidant power of this citrus refresher.

1 ORANGE
1 GRAPEFRUIT
½ CUP FIRMLY PACKED SPINACH
½ LIME
10 MINT LEAVES (OPTIONAL)

Process all ingredients in your juicer and drink immediately for the best nutritional value. You can also store this juice in an airtight container in the refrigerator for up to 3 days.

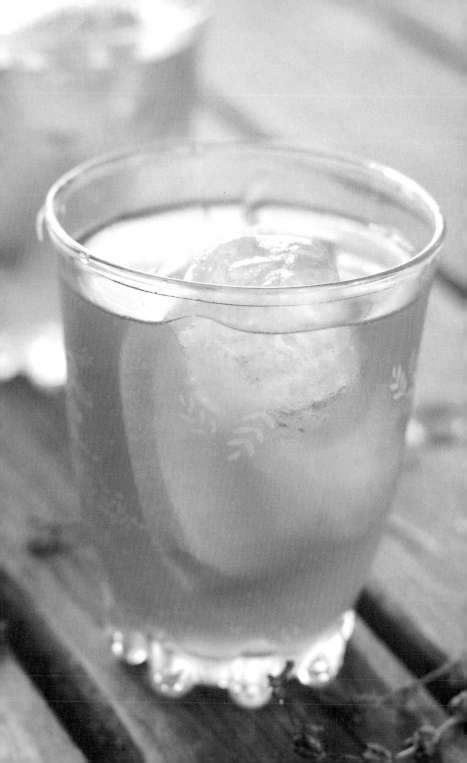

CLEANSING JUICES

TOMATO-CARROT

NUTRITIONAL VALUES 60 CALORIES / 0G FAT / 1G PROTEIN

14G CARBS / 7G SUGAR / 40MG SODIUM

JUICER TYPE

*This is a great cleansing juice if you don't have a juicer that can
handle leafy greens—and it makes a tasty mid-morning treat. The
tomatoes and carrots are packed with nutrients and also impart a
sweet, rich flavor. The lemon gives the juice a lightly tart finish.*

2 TOMATOES

2 CARROTS

2 CELERY STALKS

½ RED BELL PEPPER

½ LEMON

Process all ingredients in your juicer and drink immediately
for the best nutritional value. You can also store this juice in
an airtight container in the refrigerator for up to 3 days.

*Top cleansing foods. Since most fresh fruits and vegetables
are good for cleansing the body, most of the juices in this book can
play a beneficial role in your cleansing program (just avoid juices
that get almost all their calories from sugars). Apples, beets,
berries, cabbage, celery, grapefruit, garlic, kale, lemon, and
watercress are often cited as some of the most cleansing fruits
and vegetables.*

POWER CLEANSE

NUTRITIONAL VALUES 60 CALORIES / 1G FAT / 4G PROTEIN

12G CARBS / 6G SUGAR / 15MG SODIUM

JUICER TYPE

This cleansing juice provides a strong kick and should be a part of any cleansing ritual. Asparagus gives you protein and micronutrients, while the tomato and cucumber provide plentiful nutrients and help regulate blood sugar. Because this is one of the lower-calorie juices, you should drink it no more than once per day.

2 ASPARAGUS SPEARS
1 TOMATO
1 CUCUMBER
1 LIME
½-INCH PIECE OF GINGER

Process all ingredients in your juicer and drink immediately for the best nutritional value. You can also store this juice in an airtight container in the refrigerator for up to 3 days.

FRUITY CLEANSE

NUTRITIONAL VALUES 160 CALORIES / 3G FAT / 1G PROTEIN

20G CARBS / 10G SUGAR / 2MG SODIUM

JUICER TYPE

*This mostly fruit juice marks a sweet change of pace when you
can't bear the thought of any more vegetables. Remember that
a key reason so many vegetables are used in cleanses is to keep
sugar intake low, so indulge in this juice no more than once or
twice a week. That said, this juice packs a powerful vitamin punch
that will contribute to improved liver function and bladder health.*

3 APPLES
1 CUP CHOPPED WATERMELON
1 KIWI
½ LEMON
1 CUP STRAWBERRIES

Process all ingredients in your juicer and drink immediately
for the best nutritional value. You can also store this juice in
an airtight container in the refrigerator for up to 3 days.

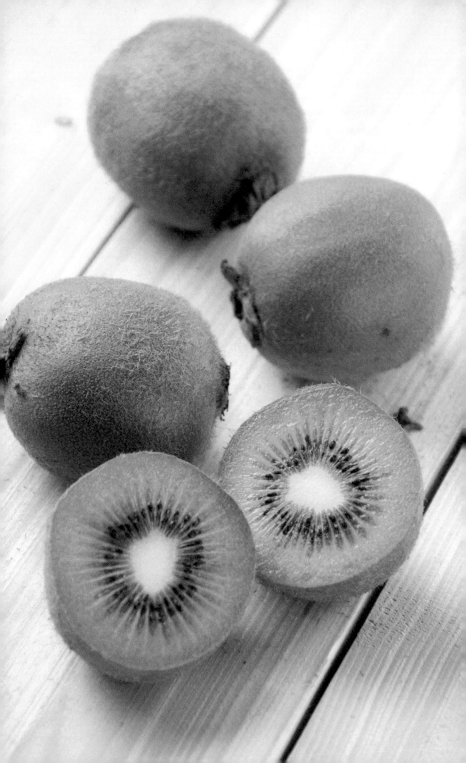

GREEN LEMONADE

NUTRITIONAL VALUES   100 CALORIES / 1G FAT / 6G PROTEIN

5G CARBS / 4G SUGAR / 3MG SODIUM

JUICER TYPE

This juice serves as the workhorse for any cleansing routine. It provides all the benefits of leafy greens, combined with sweet apple and the bright tartness of lemon. Romaine lettuce works as a solid base, providing high levels of vitamin A, folate, and essential minerals. Romaine lettuce is also a great source of complete protein. Because of the low sugar content of the other ingredients, choose a sweeter variety of apple, like McIntosh.

½ HEAD ROMAINE LETTUCE
½ CUP FIRMLY PACKED KALE
1 APPLE
½ LEMON
½-INCH PIECE OF GINGER

Process all ingredients in your juicer and drink immediately for the best nutritional value. You can also store this juice in an airtight container in the refrigerator for up to 3 days.

LEMONADE CLEANSING AID

NUTRITIONAL VALUES 110 CALORIES / 0G FAT / 0G PROTEIN

27G CARBS / 26G SUGAR / 5MG SODIUM

JUICER TYPE NONE NEEDED

Many cleansing regimens include a lemonade-style juice drink as part of their daily routines. While ingredients and schedules vary, this recipe provides the basic juice that will complement most cleansing regimens. A key to remember is to use only fresh lemon juice (not from a bottle or concentrate).

1 LEMON
1 CUP CHILLED WATER (PREFERABLY FILTERED)
2 TABLESPOONS PURE MAPLE SYRUP
⅛ TEASPOON CAYENNE PEPPER

Juice the lemon, preferably with a citrus juicer. Combine the juice with the water, maple syrup, and cayenne and stir until blended well. Drink immediately, or store in an airtight container in the refrigerator for up to 3 days.

GREEN AND ORANGE

NUTRITIONAL VALUES   120 CALORIES / 2G FAT / 3G PROTEIN

23G CARBS / 15G SUGAR / 15MG SODIUM

JUICER TYPE

This juice sticks with the cleansing theme while also offering a sweet treat. The vitamin C–packed oranges in this juice provide a wonderful burst of flavor while also strengthening your immune system. This a great juice for starting the day, or when you need to recharge in the afternoon.

>   2 ORANGES
>   ½ HEAD GREEN LEAF LETTUCE
>   ½ CUP ALFALFA SPROUTS
>   ½ CUP FIRMLY PACKED SPINACH

Process all ingredients in your juicer and drink immediately for the best nutritional value. You can also store this juice in an airtight container in the refrigerator for up to 3 days.

Cleansing booster. *Flaxseed oil is a great source of omega-3 fatty acids, which are essential for good health. This healthful oil also aids in many of the cleansing functions in the body. You can stir a half teaspoon or so of flaxseed oil into any juice without altering the flavor.*

CLEANSING PICK-ME-UP

NUTRITIONAL VALUES   130 CALORIES / 2G FAT / 2G PROTEIN

14G CARBS / 7G SUGAR / 0MG SODIUM

JUICER TYPE

*When the early stages of a juice cleanse start to become difficult,
this is a great juice to help get you over the hump. The carrots
and beets provide needed energy from complex carbohydrates,
vitamins, and minerals, and the ginger helps reduce inflammation
while providing a nice jolt to get your energy levels back up.*

3 CARROTS
½ RED BEET
1 TOMATO
1 CUCUMBER
½ LEMON
½-INCH PIECE OF GINGER

Process all ingredients in your juicer and drink immediately
for the best nutritional value. You can also store this juice in
an airtight container in the refrigerator for up to 3 days.

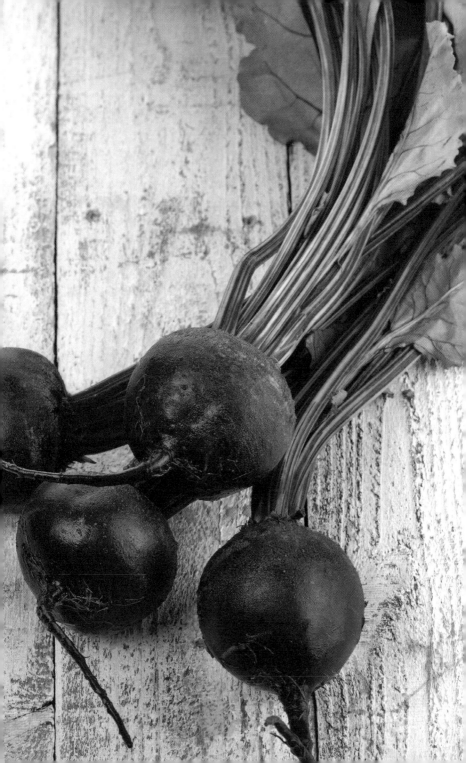

BEET, APPLE, AND MINT

NUTRITIONAL VALUES   140 CALORIES / 0G FAT / 1G PROTEIN

34G CARBS / 24G SUGAR / 10MG SODIUM

JUICER TYPE

Red beets are antioxidant superstars. They contain betalains, compounds that fight inflammation and support your detox. Betalains neutralize toxins by making them water soluble, so that they are easily flushed from the body. While the peels are also packed with nutrition, they often add a strong earthy flavor to juices. However, if you don't mind the taste, you can simply scrub and use whole beets.

    1 RED BEET
    5 CARROTS
    1 APPLE
    ¼ CUP FIRMLY PACKED MINT LEAVES

Process all ingredients in your juicer and drink immediately for the best nutritional value. You can also store this juice in an airtight container in the refrigerator for up to 3 days.

Cleansing diet challenges. *Following a juice cleanse can result in a number of unpleasant symptoms, particularly in the first day or two. Common experiences include headaches, fatigue, nausea, increased anxiety, weakness, and insomnia. As with any change in diet, it is advisable to consult a health care professional before beginning any new diet or health regimen.*

CABBAGE–CARROT

NUTRITIONAL VALUES 150 CALORIES / 1G FAT / 4G PROTEIN

30G CARBS / 20G SUGAR / 80MG SODIUM

JUICER TYPE   Ⓣ

*Cabbage is a great full-body cleanser. Its juice is rich in com-
pounds called indoles. Recent studies have shown that indoles
have cleansing properties and may even help prevent colon cancer.
When prepping romaine lettuce for juicing, it's easiest to cut it
lengthwise so you can just add the entire piece to your juicer's feed
tube without chopping.*

> 2 CUPS SLICED GREEN CABBAGE
> ½ HEAD ROMAINE LETTUCE
> 2 CARROTS

Process all ingredients in your juicer and drink immediately
for the best nutritional value. You can also store this juice in
an airtight container in the refrigerator for up to 2 days.

GREEN CLEANSE

NUTRITIONAL VALUES 170 CALORIES / 3G FAT / 3G PROTEIN

28G CARBS / 16G SUGAR / 5MG SODIUM

JUICER TYPE

One popular way of jump-starting a cleanse is with this green cleansing juice. The ingredients in this juice, particularly the beet, parsley, and endive, are known to improve liver and gallbladder function, which may aid in preventing gallstones. Adding the apple makes the juice taste a bit more pleasant, and supports healthy liver function.

1 RED BEET
¼ CUP FIRMLY PACKED PARSLEY
1 SMALL BUNCH ENDIVE
½ APPLE
1 CELERY STALK
½ LEMON

Process all ingredients in your juicer and drink immediately for the best nutritional value. You can also store this juice in an airtight container in the refrigerator for up to 3 days.

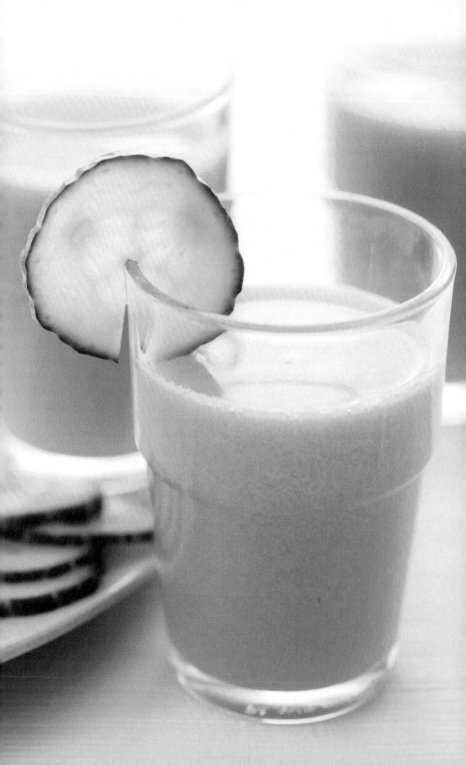

DIABETES-FRIENDLY JUICES

SPEAR AND SQUASH

NUTRITIONAL VALUES 70 CALORIES / 0G FAT / 7G PROTEIN

10G CARBS / 1G SUGAR / 120MG SODIUM

JUICER TYPE

Summer squash is high in vitamins A, B₆, and C; niacin; and water but low in sugar, making it a great vegetable to use when you need to keep your sugar intake low. Asparagus is high in protein and helps regulate blood sugar levels.

5 ASPARAGUS SPEARS
1 LARGE SUMMER SQUASH

Process all ingredients in your juicer and drink immediately for the best nutritional value. You can also store this juice in an airtight container in the refrigerator for up to 3 days.

Important information for people with diabetes. Whenever starting any new diet regimen, and especially when managing a chronic condition such as diabetes, consult your doctor to determine your dietary needs and restrictions.

ESSENTIAL MINERAL INFUSION

NUTRITIONAL VALUES   70 CALORIES / 1G FAT / 4G PROTEIN

12G CARBS / 3G SUGAR / 70MG SODIUM

JUICER TYPE

Manganese, zinc, sodium, and iron are all important minerals in a healthy diabetic diet. The ingredients in this juice provide a strong infusion of the essential minerals you need every day—as well as garlic, which is known to reduce blood sugar. This juice also helps maintain electrolyte and hydration levels and healthy blood pressure.

> 1 CUP CHOPPED BROCCOLI
> 2 CELERY STALKS
> ½ CUP FIRMLY PACKED PARSLEY
> 1 LEMON
> 1 CUCUMBER
> 2 GARLIC CLOVES

Process all ingredients in your juicer and drink immediately for the best nutritional value. You can also store this juice in an airtight container in the refrigerator for up to 2 days.

DIABETES–FRIENDLY FRUIT JUICE

NUTRITIONAL VALUES 80 CALORIES / OG FAT / 2G PROTEIN

18G CARBS / 8G SUGAR / 10MG SODIUM

JUICER TYPE

Fruit juices pack a lot of sugar per ounce. This juice dilutes the sugar content while maintaining the fruity flavor. Even so, be sure to monitor your blood sugar levels and keep the consumption of any fruit-filled juices to a moderate level. In addition to being tasty, this juice is a good source of antioxidants, especially vita-mins A, C, and E and zinc, and it contains ingredients that act as natural, gentle diuretics, which can help regulate blood pressure.

        2 CARROTS
        1 APPLE
        1 CUCUMBER
        3 ROMAINE LETTUCE LEAVES
        ½ LEMON

Process all ingredients in your juicer and drink immediately for the best nutritional value. You can also store this juice in an airtight container in the refrigerator for up to 3 days.

ZINGY CUCUMBER

NUTRITIONAL VALUES 70 CALORIES / 0G FAT / 3G PROTEIN

18G CARBS / 7G SUGAR / 20MG SODIUM

JUICER TYPE

Cucumbers and lemons are mild natural diuretics, which help regulate blood pressure. This juice is also light and refreshing and packs a little zip, making it a great refreshment on a sunny day. A pinch of salt will not only bring out the flavor but also fortify your diet with added electrolytes.

2 CUCUMBERS
½ LEMON
½-INCH PIECE OF GINGER
PINCH OF SALT (OPTIONAL)

Process the first three ingredients in your juicer; stir in the salt if desired. Drink this juice immediately for the best nutritional value, or store in an airtight container in the refrigerator for up to 3 days.

VITAMIN E VEGGIE SUPPLEMENT

NUTRITIONAL VALUES   80 CALORIES / 1G FAT / 5G PROTEIN

15G CARBS / 6G SUGAR / 90MG SODIUM

JUICER TYPE

Staying healthy while managing diabetes generally requires an increased vitamin intake. Maintaining a high vitamin E intake can decrease the amount of insulin needed to help control diabetes, while also providing numerous other health benefits. All the ingredients in this juice are good sources of vitamin E. When mixed together, these particular veggies are also tasty and balanced in sugar.

3 TOMATOES
2 CARROTS
½ CUP FIRMLY PACKED WATERCRESS
½ CUP FIRMLY PACKED SPINACH

Process all ingredients in your juicer and drink immediately for the best nutritional value. You can also store this juice in an airtight container in the refrigerator for up to 3 days.

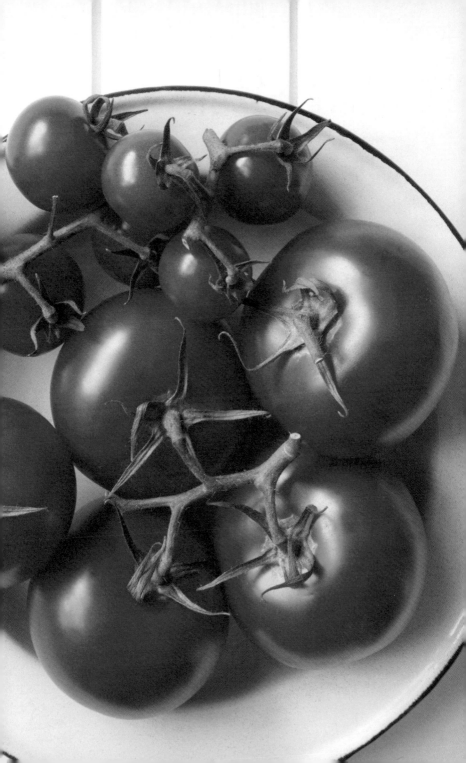

GARDEN VEGETABLE JUICE FOR REDUCING DIABETES

NUTRITIONAL VALUES 110 CALORIES / 0G FAT / 7G PROTEIN

20G CARBS / 7G SUGAR / 20MG SODIUM

JUICER TYPE

This juice is high in manganese, which is important for regulating blood glucose levels. Its ingredients are also rich in other minerals, including zinc and calcium, which are especially important when following a diabetic eating plan.

1 TOMATO
2 CELERY STALKS
⅓ CUP CHOPPED BROCCOLI
1 GARLIC CLOVE
3 KALE LEAVES

Process all ingredients in your juicer and drink immediately for the best nutritional value. You can also store this juice in an airtight container in the refrigerator for up to 2 days.

SWEET SPROUTS
AND BEANS

NUTRITIONAL VALUES   120 CALORIES / 1G FAT / 8G PROTEIN

30G CARBS / 3G SUGAR / 40MG SODIUM

JUICER TYPE

*Sprouts offer so many health benefits that you really can't go
wrong getting more of them in your diet. This juice in particular
offers up nutrients and minerals to help you maintain steady
blood sugar levels while also supplying you with protein and
complex carbs. It's an excellent meal replacement.*

> ½ CUP ALFALFA SPROUTS
> 1 CUP BRUSSELS SPROUTS
> 1 CUP GREEN BEANS
> 1 LIME

Process all ingredients in your juicer and drink immediately
for the best nutritional value. You can also store this juice in
an airtight container in the refrigerator for up to 2 days.

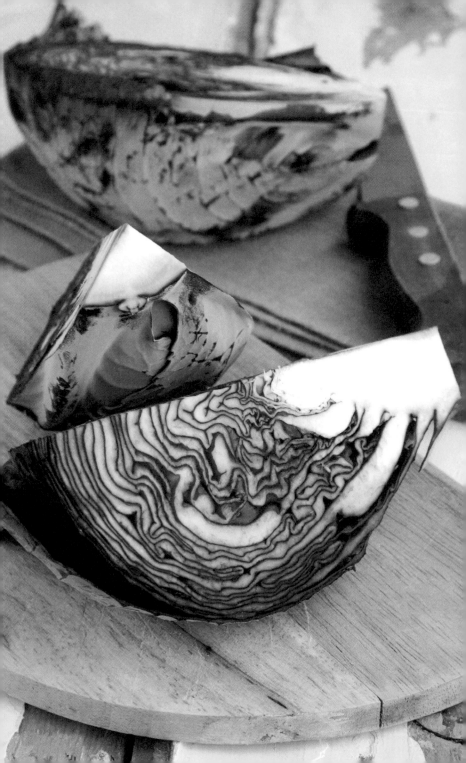

APPLE, CABBAGE, AND CARROT

NUTRITIONAL VALUES   120 CALORIES / 1G FAT / 2G PROTEIN

29G CARBS / 19G SUGAR / 25MG SODIUM

JUICER TYPE

Cabbages are inexpensive and fantastic for helping you maintain proper blood sugar. They have one of the lowest glycemic indexes of all produce and are great sources of vitamins B_6 and C. Low-carb cabbage also helps dilute the more sugar-laden carrots and apples to a safe level, while still contributing essential nutrients needed to help control diabetes, especially vitamin E. Purple cabbage is preferred for its high levels of vitamin A, but any variety is fine.

½ HEAD PURPLE CABBAGE
1 APPLE
1 CARROT

Process all ingredients in your juicer and drink immediately for the best nutritional value. You can also store this juice in an airtight container in the refrigerator for up to 2 days.

GREEN-SPIKED ORANGE JUICE

NUTRITIONAL VALUES   150 CALORIES / 1G FAT / 6G PROTEIN

38G CARBS / 25G SUGAR / 25MG SODIUM

JUICER TYPE

The high sugar level of the oranges is complemented by the more complex nutrition profile of the greens, making this a healthful, mildly sweet juice to start the day. If you are using a centrifugal juicer, you can replace the kale with an additional stalk of broccoli.

2 ORANGES
⅓ CUP CHOPPED BROCCOLI
3 KALE LEAVES

Process all ingredients in your juicer and drink immediately for the best nutritional value. You can also store this juice in an airtight container in the refrigerator for up to 3 days.

CARROT, BROCCOLI, AND CAULIFLOWER

NUTRITIONAL VALUES 180 CALORIES / 1G FAT / 7G PROTEIN

48G CARBS / 22G SUGAR / 150MG SODIUM

JUICER TYPE

*The American Diabetes Association recommends that people
with diabetes get as many of their carbohydrates as possible from
whole fruits and vegetables. The high fiber and complex carbo-
hydrate content of this juice is digested much more slowly than
starchy, sugar-laden processed foods.*

    4 CARROTS
    ¾ CUP CHOPPED CAULIFLOWER
    ¾ CUP CHOPPED BROCCOLI
    1 CELERY STALK
    ½ LEMON

Process all ingredients in your juicer and drink immediately
for the best nutritional value. You can also store this juice in
an airtight container in the refrigerator for up to 2 days.

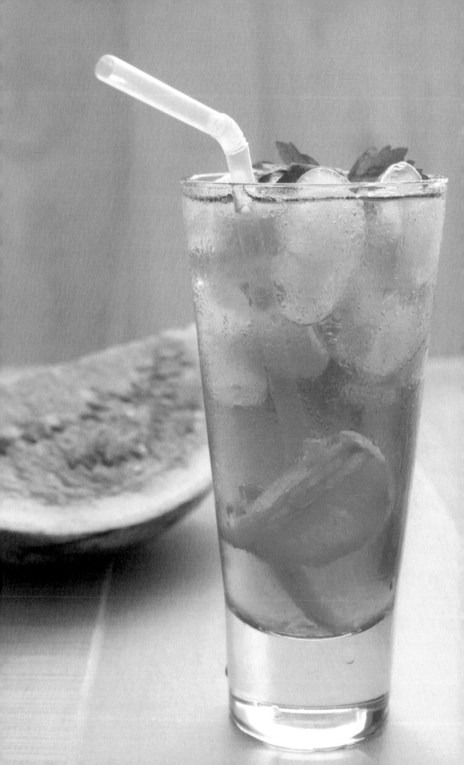

10

DIGESTIVE HEALTH JUICES

WATERMELON–MINT

NUTRITIONAL VALUES 80 CALORIES / 0G FAT / 1G PROTEIN

19G CARBS / 15G SUGAR / 2MG SODIUM

JUICER TYPE

*Mint has long been used to relieve bloating, gas, and other diges-
tive health issues and discomforts. Watermelon is gentle on the
stomach and a great source of potassium, which can help maintain stomach acid levels. If this juice is too sweet for your taste,
replace half the watermelon with a seeded cucumber.*

10 MINT LEAVES
3 CUPS CHOPPED WATERMELON

Using a muddler or wooden spoon, crush the mint leaves in
the bottom of a glass, and then add a few ice cubes. Process the
watermelon in your juicer, add to the glass, stir well, and enjoy.

CARROT–GINGER

NUTRITIONAL VALUES 80 CALORIES / 0G FAT / 1G PROTEIN

19G CARBS / 12G SUGAR / 5MG SODIUM

JUICER TYPE

For centuries, ginger has been used for a wide variety of ailments, especially those related to digestive health. This rhizome has been shown to provide relief from diarrhea, upset stomach, and nausea. Carrots have a soothing, gentle sweet flavor that can relieve anxiety, often the cause of stomach ailments.

    3 CARROTS
    1 APPLE
    1–INCH PIECE OF GINGER

Process all ingredients in your juicer and drink immediately for the best nutritional value. You can also store this juice in an airtight container in the refrigerator for up to 3 days.

Medicinal ginger. *Ginger has been used as a natural remedy for centuries. In fact, many modern antacids, laxatives, and anti-gas medications are based on or use compounds found in ginger. Ginger has also been found to relieve nausea both from motion sickness and related to pregnancy.*

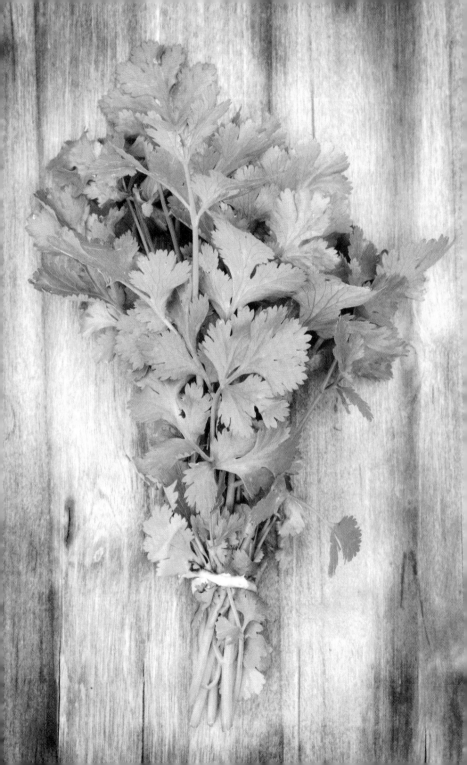

CILANTRO AND GINGER GI RELIEF

NUTRITIONAL VALUES   80 CALORIES / 1G FAT / 0G PROTEIN

17G CARBS / 6G SUGAR / 70MG SODIUM

JUICER TYPE

Cilantro is one of the best herbs for cleansing the digestive system, helping remove heavy metals from the body, and even relieving symptoms of mild food-borne illnesses. The electrolytes found in celery and apples can also help you recover from stomach ailments such as diarrhea.

1½ CUPS FIRMLY PACKED CILANTRO
1-INCH PIECE OF GINGER
4 CELERY STALKS
1 APPLE
½ LIME

Process all ingredients in your juicer and drink immediately for the best nutritional value. You can also store this juice in an airtight container in the refrigerator for up to 3 days.

BLOAT RELIEF

NUTRITIONAL VALUES 85 CALORIES / 1G FAT / 2G PROTEIN

18G CARBS / 10G SUGAR / 27MG SODIUM

JUICER TYPE

The ingredients in this juice provide high levels of pectin, which has been shown to be good for colon health. In addition, cucumbers contain erepsin, an enzyme that aids in the digestion of proteins (which can often cause feelings of bloat). Finally, apple and cucumber have gentle laxative properties, which can help kick-start your system.

    1 CUCUMBER
    2 APPLES
    2 CARROTS
    ½ LEMON

Process all ingredients in your juicer and drink immediately for the best nutritional value. You can also store this juice in an airtight container in the refrigerator for up to 3 days.

GINGER, APPLE, CARROT, AND PINEAPPLE

NUTRITIONAL VALUES 100 CALORIES / 0G FAT / 1G PROTEIN

24G CARBS / 19G SUGAR / 10MG SODIUM

JUICER TYPE

Many proteins, particularly those from animal sources, are difficult to digest and can cause a number of health discomforts. Pineapple contains an enzyme that attacks proteins, breaking them up into simpler forms. This is one reason pineapple juice is often used as a marinade for tenderizing meats.

1 APPLE
2 CARROTS
1 CUP CHOPPED PINEAPPLE
½-INCH PIECE OF GINGER

Process all ingredients in your juicer and drink immediately for the best nutritional value. You can also store this juice in an airtight container in the refrigerator for up to 3 days.

SOOTHING STOMACH
FRUIT JUICE

NUTRITIONAL VALUES 100 CALORIES / 1G FAT / 2G PROTEIN

22G CARBS / 17G SUGAR / 10MG SODIUM

JUICER TYPE

*Lemon and ginger are both natural remedies that can soothe
many stomachaches and pains. This recipe typically is very effec-
tive for stomach pains related to stress or eating too heavy a meal.
However, if you are experiencing indigestion, high-acid foods like
lemons and oranges can make it worse, so proceed with caution.*

1 APPLE
1 ORANGE
1 CUP FIRMLY PACKED SPINACH
1 CELERY STALK
½ LEMON
½-INCH PIECE OF GINGER

Process all ingredients in your juicer and drink immediately
for the best nutritional value. You can also store this juice in
an airtight container in the refrigerator for up to 3 days.

APPLE, STRAWBERRY, AND MINT

NUTRITIONAL VALUES   100 CALORIES / 0G FAT / 1G PROTEIN

24G CARBS / 20G SUGAR / 10MG SODIUM

JUICER TYPE

In cases of mild food poisoning or other upset-stomach symptoms, mint can provide nearly instant relief. Apples can also aid digestion with their mild laxative effect, helping clean out the body's digestive system. For best results when juicing, toss the mint leaves and strawberries together so they are well mixed when added to the machine.

>   1 APPLE
>   1½ CUPS STRAWBERRIES
>   ¼ CUP FIRMLY PACKED MINT LEAVES

Process all ingredients in your juicer and drink immediately for the best nutritional value. You can also store this juice in an airtight container in the refrigerator for up to 3 days.

PEAR AND APPLE

NUTRITIONAL VALUES   120 CALORIES / 0G FAT / 1G PROTEIN

24G CARBS / 17G SUGAR / 5MG SODIUM

JUICER TYPE

Pears and apples are both mild laxatives, and juicing removes much of the insoluble fiber that can cause feelings of bloat. What's left is a gentle intestinal cleanser high in electrolytes and vitamins. These fruits are also high in pectin and soluble fiber, both critical for colon health.

2 PEARS
1 APPLE
1 LEMON WEDGE

Process all ingredients in your juicer and drink immediately for the best nutritional value. You can also store this juice in an airtight container in the refrigerator for up to 3 days.

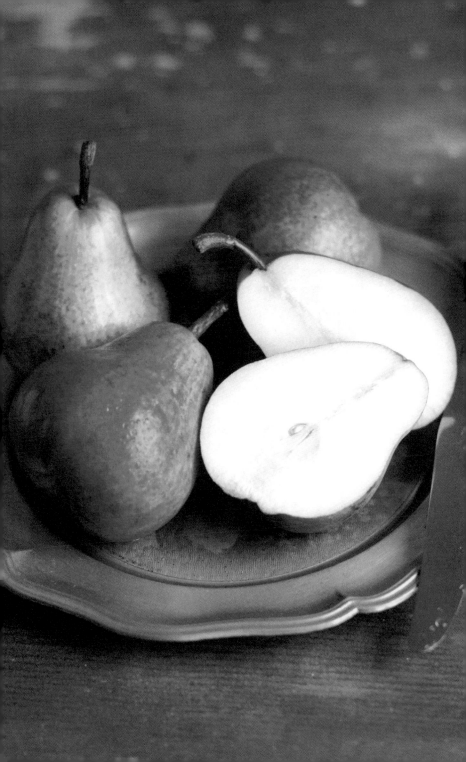

TROPICAL DIGESTIVE AID

NUTRITIONAL VALUES   130 CALORIES / 0G FAT / 2G PROTEIN

30G CARBS / 23G SUGAR / 5MG SODIUM

JUICER TYPE

Both papaya and pineapple contain protein-busting enzymes that can aid in digestion, relieve feelings of bloat, and reduce gas. Bodybuilders and athletes on intense training regimens often supplement their diets with these fruits.

1 CUP CHOPPED PAPAYA
1 CUP CHOPPED PINEAPPLE
1 ORANGE

Process all ingredients in your juicer and drink immediately for the best nutritional value. You can also store this juice in an airtight container in the refrigerator for up to 3 days.

PINEAPPLE AND PEAR COOLER

NUTRITIONAL VALUES 130 CALORIES / 0G FAT / 1G PROTEIN

32G CARBS / 25G SUGAR / 7MG SODIUM

JUICER TYPE

Pears contain numerous compounds healthful for the colon and the body's digestive system as a whole. Pineapple aids in the digestion of proteins that can cause a number of digestive discomforts. Finally, mint can soothe an upset stomach. Combined, these ingredients make a great overall tonic for digestive relief and health.

    2 CUPS CHOPPED PINEAPPLE
    1 PEAR
    ¼ CUP FIRMLY PACKED MINT LEAVES

Process all ingredients in your juicer and drink immediately for the best nutritional value. You can also store this juice in an airtight container in the refrigerator for up to 3 days.

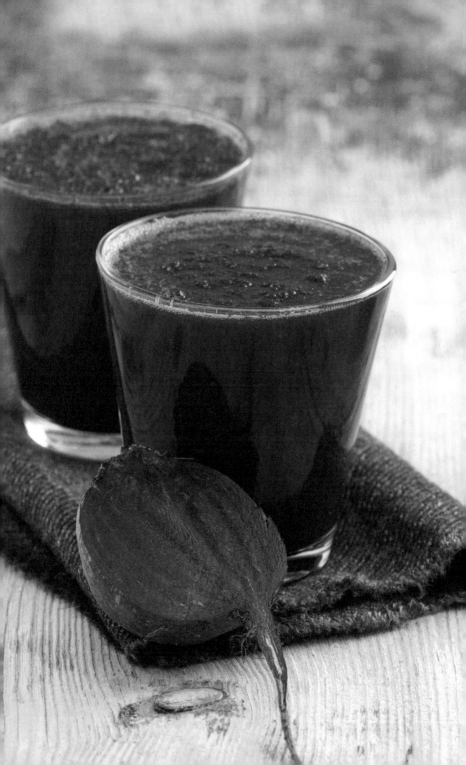

11

HIGH-ENERGY JUICES

THE CURE FOR WHAT KALES YOU

NUTRITIONAL VALUES 40 CALORIES / 0G FAT / 2G PROTEIN

8G CARBS / 6G SUGAR / 40MG SODIUM

JUICER TYPE

This energizing juice is packed with chlorophyll, which provides an all-natural energy boost. The addition of beets and apples provides readily accessible energy and a delicious light sweetness. This is a perfect preworkout drink to help you get motivated.

4 OR 5 KALE LEAVES
1 RED BEET, INCLUDING GREENS
1 APPLE
½ CUP FIRMLY PACKED SPINACH
¼ CUP FIRMLY PACKED PARSLEY
½ LEMON

Process all ingredients in your juicer and drink immediately for the best nutritional value. You can also store this juice in an airtight container in the refrigerator for up to 3 days.

SUPER ENERGY AND METABOLISM BOOST

NUTRITIONAL VALUES   50 CALORIES / 0G FAT / 2G PROTEIN

10G CARBS / 7G SUGAR / 40MG SODIUM

JUICER TYPE

The ingredients in this juice all have metabolism-boosting proper-ties in addition to providing a nice energy boost on their own. Combine that with the minerals and electrolytes from the parsley and lemon, and you have a juice that will not only get you ener-gized but also keep you going throughout the day.

1 CUP FIRMLY PACKED PARSLEY
½ LEMON
1 APPLE
2 CARROTS
2-INCH PIECE OF GINGER
1 RED CHILE PEPPER (SUCH AS SERRANO)

Process all ingredients in your juicer and drink immediately for the best nutritional value. You can also store this juice in an airtight container in the refrigerator for up to three days.

The metabolic power of juice. *The process of juicing breaks down cell walls, creating a food from which nutrients and min-erals are readily accessible. This allows the body to absorb more nutrients quickly, often resulting in feelings of increased energy and alertness.*

JET LAG TONIC

NUTRITIONAL VALUES   50 CALORIES / 0G FAT / 2G PROTEIN

12G CARBS / 3G SUGAR / 40MG SODIUM

JUICER TYPE

Celery and romaine have calming properties that can aid in providing you with restful sleep. Drinking this juice after a major time zone change will help you reset your internal clock. To make this juice in a centrifugal juicer, bunch the parsley into a tight ball, and feed it into the juicer sandwiched between stalks of celery.

    4 CELERY STALKS
    ½ HEAD ROMAINE LETTUCE
    ¼ CUP FIRMLY PACKED PARSLEY
    ½ LEMON

Process all ingredients in your juicer and drink immediately for the best nutritional value. You can also store this juice in an airtight container in the refrigerator for up to 3 days.

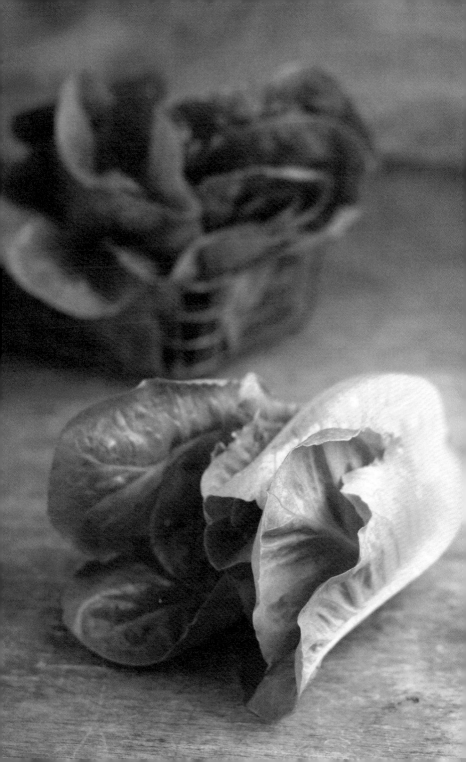

THE BEETS GO ON

NUTRITIONAL VALUES 80 CALORIES / 0G FAT / 2G PROTEIN

19G CARBS / 10G SUGAR / 65MG SODIUM

JUICER TYPE

Packed with both complex and accessible carbohydrates, beet juice is like rocket fuel for the body. Containing simple carbohydrates for instant energy as well as complex carbohydrates and electrolytes for endurance, this juice makes a great alternative to coffee for an afternoon boost.

    1 RED BEET
    1 APPLE
    2 CARROTS
    ½ CUCUMBER

Process all ingredients in your juicer and drink immediately for the best nutritional value. You can also store this juice in an airtight container in the refrigerator for up to 3 days.

RUNNER'S FRIEND
ENERGY DRINK

NUTRITIONAL VALUES   70 CALORIES / 0G FAT / 2G PROTEIN

16G CARBS / 5G SUGAR / 5MG SODIUM

JUICER TYPE

Powerful enough to help you burn through the most intense work-outs, this juice is full of phytonutrients. Purple cabbage contains energizing vitamins C and B to boost your metabolism, while cucumbers serve as a refreshing, nutritious base full of electrolytes essential for maintaining healthy hydration. The grapes also provide a bit of energy, and an added sweetness.

½ HEAD PURPLE CABBAGE
1 CUCUMBER
¼ CUP RED GRAPES
1 APPLE
PINCH OF SALT (OPTIONAL)

Process the first four ingredients in your juicer; stir in the salt if desired. Drink this juice immediately for the best nutritional value, or store in an airtight container in the refrigerator for up to 2 days.

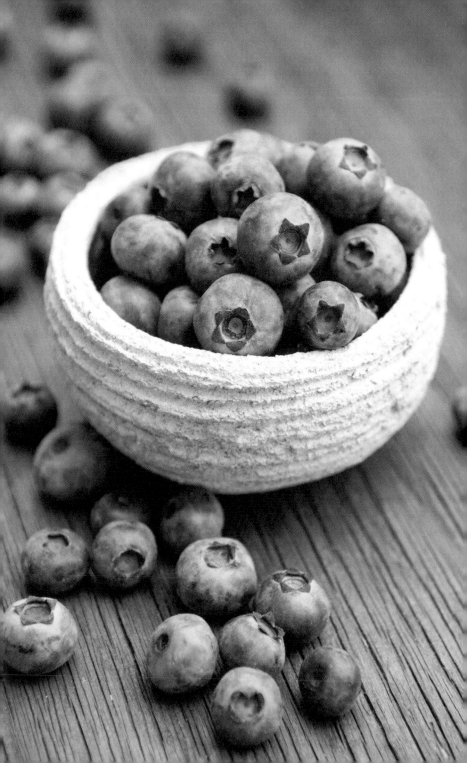

FATIGUE RELIEF

NUTRITIONAL VALUES   80 CALORIES / 1G FAT / 4G PROTEIN

16G CARBS / 5G SUGAR / 90MG SODIUM

JUICER TYPE

A common cause of fatigue is not having enough folate in your diet. Flaxseed oil is one of the best sources of folate, but the nutrient is also found in abundance in broccoli and cauliflower, making this juice a great choice with or without the optional supplement. Blueberries have also been shown to relieve the symptoms of chronic fatigue syndrome in some individuals.

>   1 CUP CHOPPED BROCCOLI
>   1 CUP CHOPPED CAULIFLOWER
>   1 CUP BLUEBERRIES
>   1 TEASPOON FLAXSEED OIL (OPTIONAL)

Process all ingredients in your juicer; stir in oil if desired. Drink immediately for the best nutritional value. You can also store this juice in an airtight container in the refrigerator for up to 2 days.

All-day metabolic boost. Check out Chapter 3, Breakfast Juices; Chapter 4, Brain-Nourishing Juices; and Chapter 6, Anti-Aging Juices for additional juices that help build and maintain a healthy metabolism from morning to night.

SLEEP AID FOR AN ENERGETIC MORNING

NUTRITIONAL VALUES 90 CALORIES / 1G FAT / 3G PROTEIN

20G CARBS / 7G SUGAR / 60MG SODIUM

JUICER TYPE

Nothing can compare to the energy you get from a good night's rest. Romaine lettuce has been shown to have an amazing ability to help people fall asleep and sleep more restfully. Celery and carrots also help soothe the body and mind, alleviating stress and strain after a busy day.

½ HEAD ROMAINE LETTUCE
2 CELERY STALKS
2 CARROTS

Process all ingredients in your juicer and drink immediately for the best nutritional value. You can also store this juice in an airtight container in the refrigerator for up to 3 days.

CITRUS ENERGY

NUTRITIONAL VALUES   90 CALORIES / OG FAT / 1G PROTEIN

22G CARBS / 18G SUGAR / 5MG SODIUM

JUICER TYPE

Citrus fruits are great sources of energy and vitamin C. Their juices are the original sports drinks, and this juice blend packs a great punch. Grapefruit is a powerful metabolism enhancer and a great source of potassium and folate. Together, these two nutrients provide energy and help the body maintain proper hydration. Oranges add sweetness, and the lemon gives a little extra zing.

> 1 GRAPEFRUIT
> 2 ORANGES
> 1 LEMON

Process all ingredients in your juicer and drink immediately for the best nutritional value. You can also store this juice in an airtight container in the refrigerator for up to 3 days.

ENERGY BOOST

NUTRITIONAL VALUES   90 CALORIES / 0G FAT / 1G PROTEIN

21G CARBS / 17G SUGAR / 2MG SODIUM

JUICER TYPE

This juice is less about flavor and more about getting an energy boost to rival coffee or any sports drink. While healthy on its own, the pineapple is mainly there to make the whole thing go down more smoothly, so feel free to leave it out and down the rest as a shot.

1 CUP FIRMLY PACKED WHEATGRASS
½ CUP CRANBERRIES
½ LEMON
1-INCH PIECE OF GINGER
1 CUP CHOPPED PINEAPPLE

Process all ingredients in your juicer and drink immediately for the best nutritional value. You can also store this juice in an airtight container in the refrigerator for up to 3 days.

ANEMIA BUSTER

NUTRITIONAL VALUES 100 CALORIES / 1G FAT / 2G PROTEIN

23G CARBS / 19G SUGAR / 20MG SODIUM

JUICER TYPE

Iron is essential for the blood's ability to carry oxygen, and a diet low in iron can cause anemia. Pineapple is a great source of iron and vitamin C to help power your way through the day. Spinach packs even more iron, keeping you energized while holding anemia and its related symptoms at bay. The electrolytes and minerals found in this juice will also help keep you hydrated.

1 CUP CHOPPED PINEAPPLE
½ CUP FIRMLY PACKED SPINACH
1 CUCUMBER

Process all ingredients in your juicer and drink immediately for the best nutritional value. You can also store this juice in an airtight container in the refrigerator for up to 3 days.

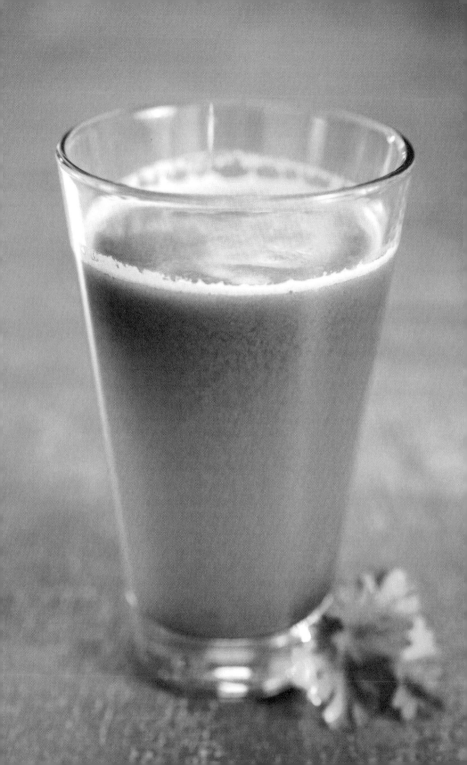

12

GREEN JUICES

GREEN AND CLEAN

NUTRITIONAL VALUES   50 CALORIES / 0G FAT / 2G PROTEIN

10G CARBS / 3G SUGAR / 50MG SODIUM

JUICER TYPE

This juice, and green juices in general, are great full-body cleansers. Packed with superfood leafy greens, this mixture offers a great way to incorporate a wide variety of nutrient-rich vegetables into your diet in a simple, easy-to-drink juice. Feel free to substitute or add small amounts of other fresh green vegetables for added variety.

> ½ HEAD ROMAINE LETTUCE
> 1 APPLE
> ½ CUP FIRMLY PACKED SPINACH
> ¾ CUP FIRMLY PACKED CILANTRO
> 1 LEMON
> 1–INCH PIECE OF GINGER

Process all ingredients in your juicer and drink immediately for the best nutritional value. You can also store this juice in an airtight container in the refrigerator for up to 3 days.

Reasons to go green. *Dark green vegetables are often extremely high in nutrient value, and simultaneously very low in calories. By incorporating green juice into your daily diet, you will help load your body with essential nutrients at levels difficult to achieve through food alone.*

GREEN DETOX

NUTRITIONAL VALUES   60 CALORIES / 0G FAT / 2G PROTEIN

14G CARBS / 6G SUGAR / 5MG SODIUM

JUICER TYPE

*Packed with cancer-fighting antioxidants, this juice provides a
quick, simple way to get a burst of vitamins and minerals from fresh
fruits and vegetables in a single glass. You can replace the grapes
with almost any sweet fruit, such as a Fuji apple or Bosc pear.*

> 1 CUP FIRMLY PACKED CILANTRO
> 1 CUCUMBER
> 1 CUP FIRMLY PACKED SPINACH
> 1 LIME
> 1 CUP RED GRAPES

Process all ingredients in your juicer and drink immediately
for the best nutritional value. You can also store this juice in
an airtight container in the refrigerator for up to 3 days.

"GREEN" APPLE

NUTRITIONAL VALUES   70 CALORIES / 0G FAT / 4G PROTEIN

14G CARBS / 7G SUGAR / 50MG SODIUM

JUICER TYPE

This juice is so delicious you'll have trouble believing it's healthy. The light, nutritious romaine complements the sweet apple, tart lime, and aromatic mint perfectly. This juice makes a great snack alternative that won't make you feel that you are sacrificing anything.

    10 MINT LEAVES
    1 APPLE
    1 HEAD ROMAINE LETTUCE
    1 LIME

In a glass, muddle the mint with a wooden spoon. Process the remaining ingredients in your juicer and mix well with the mint. Drink this juice immediately for the best nutritional value, or store in an airtight container in the refrigerator for up to 3 days.

GREEN IRON

NUTRITIONAL VALUES 70 CALORIES / 0G FAT / 4G PROTEIN

14G CARBS / 3G SUGAR / 70MG SODIUM

JUICER TYPE

Spinach is a great source of iron and many other essential nutrients, and juicing is the best way of extracting the most powerful nutritional punch from this superfood. This juice is also a great source of vitamin C, which counteracts the oxalic acid in spinach that slows down the absorption of calcium and other minerals.

2 CUPS FIRMLY PACKED SPINACH
3 KALE LEAVES
3 CELERY STALKS
½ CUCUMBER
½ LEMON
1 APPLE

Process all ingredients in your juicer and drink immediately for the best nutritional value. You can also store this juice in an airtight container in the refrigerator for up to 3 days.

Green for iron. Most green vegetables are rich sources of iron and great for helping prevent or combat iron-related anemia. Symptoms of anemia include fatigue and low energy, rapid or irregular heartbeat, headache, dizziness, and pale skin. When your parents said to eat your spinach in order to grow up healthy and strong, they weren't kidding.

CLASSIC GREEN JUICE

NUTRITIONAL VALUES 70 CALORIES / 0G FAT / 3G PROTEIN

15G CARBS / 4G SUGAR / 70MG SODIUM

JUICER TYPE

The ingredients in this recipe are most commonly used when making a generic "green juice." Packed with nutrients, this reliable concoction also helps detoxify the body. To extract as much juice as possible from the kale with a centrifugal juicer, try rolling the leaves tightly around the celery stalks.

1 CUCUMBER
2 CELERY STALKS
1 APPLE
8 TO 10 KALE LEAVES
½ LEMON
½-INCH PIECE OF GINGER

Process all ingredients in your juicer and drink immediately for the best nutritional value. You can also store this juice in an airtight container in the refrigerator for up to 3 days.

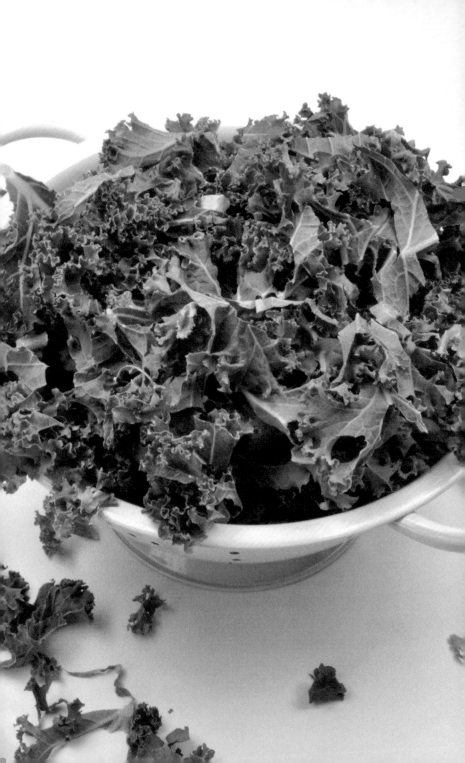

SPICY, SWEET, AND GREEN

NUTRITIONAL VALUES 70 CALORIES / 0G FAT / 2G PROTEIN

16G CARBS / 4G SUGAR / 50MG SODIUM

JUICER TYPE

Pineapple juice spiked with chile and lime makes a great summer drink. Kale and cucumber give this juice all the health benefits of a green juice without taking away its delicious fruity flavor. Chile peppers have been shown to boost metabolism, while the cucumber and kale are great sources of electrolytes. This juice will give you a quick jump start without any energy crash later on.

2 CUPS CHOPPED PINEAPPLE

1 JALAPEÑO PEPPER OR OTHER CHILE

½ LIME

4 OR 5 KALE LEAVES

½ CUCUMBER

Process all ingredients in your juicer and drink immediately for the best nutritional value. You can also store this juice in an airtight container in the refrigerator for up to 3 days.

Giving green a spin. While it is not generally recommended to juice leafy green vegetables in a centrifugal juicer, it is possible. The main issue is that centrifugal juicers will not give you the best yield of juice from what you put in. If you simply want to try a green juice without buying new equipment, you can try increasing the amount of greens you add to the juicer. You can also get decent results by rolling the leaves into a tight tube, like a rolled-up newspaper.

BASIL MOJITO

NUTRITIONAL VALUES 80 CALORIES / OG FAT / 1G PROTEIN

19G CARBS / 12G SUGAR / 90MG SODIUM

JUICER TYPE

This juice has a summery herb flavor that will remind you of its namesake cocktail. Besides being rich in antioxidants, basil also has remarkable anti-inflammatory and anti-swelling properties. It has also been found to help cleanse certain toxins found in the heart and liver. For the best flavor, select a sweeter variety of apple, such as Fuji.

10 MINT LEAVES
1 CUP FIRMLY PACKED BASIL
2 APPLES
1 CUCUMBER
1 LIME

In a large glass, muddle the mint with a wooden spoon. Process the remaining ingredients in your juicer, and pour the juice over the mint, adding ice if desired. Drink immediately for the best nutritional value, or store in an airtight container in the refrigerator for up to 3 days.

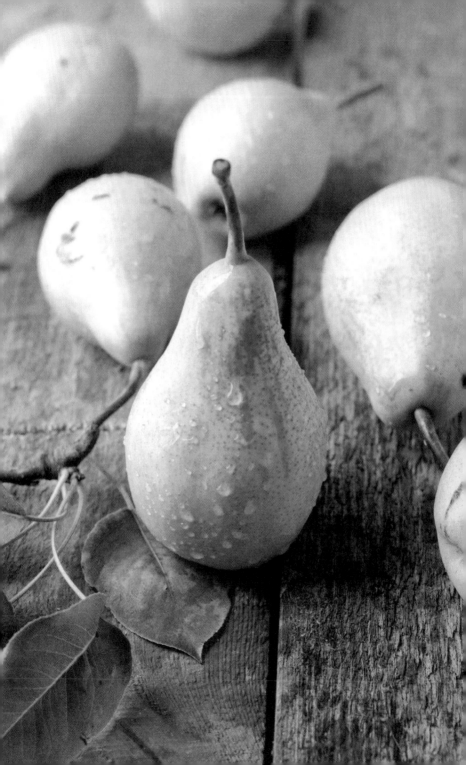

SPINACH LEMONADE

NUTRITIONAL VALUES 70 CALORIES / 0G FAT / 4G PROTEIN

14G CARBS / 5G SUGAR / 40MG SODIUM

JUICER TYPE

Here's all the refreshment of lemonade in a far healthier package!
Feel free to adjust the amount of lemon and spinach to your liking.
If you generally aren't a fan of green juices, this might be a great
entry point. You can even start with less than a cup of spinach,
gradually working your way up to let your palate adjust.

½ LEMON
2 CUPS FIRMLY PACKED SPINACH
1 APPLE
1 PEAR
1 CUCUMBER
1 TO 3 TEASPOONS AGAVE NECTAR (OPTIONAL)

Process the first five ingredients in your juicer, and sweeten
to taste with agave nectar if desired. Drink this juice immediately for the best nutritional value, or store in an airtight
container in the refrigerator for up to 3 days.

GREEN AND TART

NUTRITIONAL VALUES 80 CALORIES / 0G FAT / 2G PROTEIN

19G CARBS / 7G SUGAR / 60MG SODIUM

JUICER TYPE

This juice blends antioxidant-packed leafy greens and herbs with sweet and tangy citrus to make a healthful, low-calorie, vitamin-packed juice for any occasion. If you use a centrifugal juicer and want to incorporate spinach into your juices, a small handful of baby spinach processed with the juice in a blender until smooth does the job nicely—with an added fiber bonus.

½ HEAD ROMAINE LETTUCE
1 CUP FIRMLY PACKED SPINACH
½ CUP FIRMLY PACKED CILANTRO
3 ORANGES
1 LIME

Process all ingredients in your juicer and drink immediately for the best nutritional value. You can also store this juice in an airtight container in the refrigerator for up to 3 days.

Rinse your spinach well. Spinach grows low to the ground and has a rough texture, so a lot of dirt and grit can get stuck between the leaves. For the best results, separate all the leaves and rinse thoroughly before juicing.

GREEN OJ

NUTRITIONAL VALUES 80 CALORIES / OG FAT / 2G PROTEIN

19G CARBS / 13G SUGAR / 50MG SODIUM

JUICER TYPE

This "orange juice" (which is actually green) keeps most of that wonderful flavor while also packing in a ton of green vegetable nutrition. The celery and cucumber provide additional minerals and electrolytes, making this a great juice to help you recover from an intense workout.

2 ORANGES
1 APPLE
2 CELERY STALKS
½ CUCUMBER
1 CUP FIRMLY PACKED SPINACH

Process all ingredients in your juicer and drink immediately for the best nutritional value. You can also store this juice in an airtight container in the refrigerator for up to 3 days.

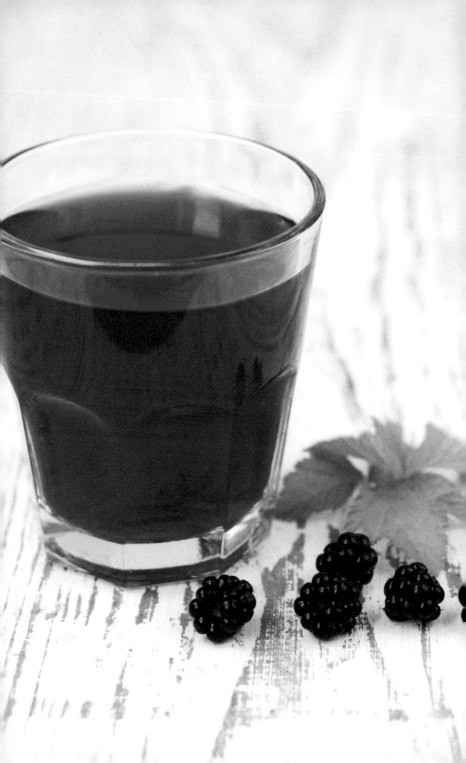

13

HEALTHFUL
SKIN JUICES

SMOOTH AND GLOWING
SKIN VEGGIE JUICE

NUTRITIONAL VALUES   60 CALORIES / 1G FAT / 4G PROTEIN

10G CARBS / 3G SUGAR / 120MG SODIUM

JUICER TYPE

Cucumbers and celery are both good sources of silica, a mineral that promotes healthy nails and skin. Silica is essential for maintaining healthy connective tissue, which helps the skin maintain its elasticity and smoothness. This juice is also a good source of zinc and healthy omega-3 fatty acids.

1 CUCUMBER
2 CELERY STALKS
1 CUP FIRMLY PACKED SPINACH
1 CUP GREEN BEANS
1 GARLIC CLOVE
½-INCH PIECE OF GINGER

Process all ingredients in your juicer and drink immediately for the best nutritional value. You can also store this juice in an airtight container in the refrigerator for up to 3 days.

Good hydration for good skin.   Hydration plays an important role in healthy-looking skin, which is why juicing is a great way to supplement your diet. In addition, the antioxidants packed into every glass of fresh juice found in this book help neutralize free radicals that cause wrinkles and other signs of aging.

BEET, CARROT, AND GINGER

NUTRITIONAL VALUES   60 CALORIES / OG FAT / 2G PROTEIN

8G CARBS / 4G SUGAR / 64MG SODIUM

JUICER TYPE

Consuming foods high in iron, such as beets, has been shown to speed the healing process and eliminate canker sores around the mouth. This juice is also high in vitamins A, B, and C. Carrots are high in beta-carotene, an antioxidant that helps repair skin tissue and protects against sun damage.

1 OR 2 RED BEETS
4 CARROTS
½-INCH PIECE OF GINGER

Process all ingredients in your juicer and drink immediately for the best nutritional value. You can also store this juice in an airtight container in the refrigerator for up to 3 days.

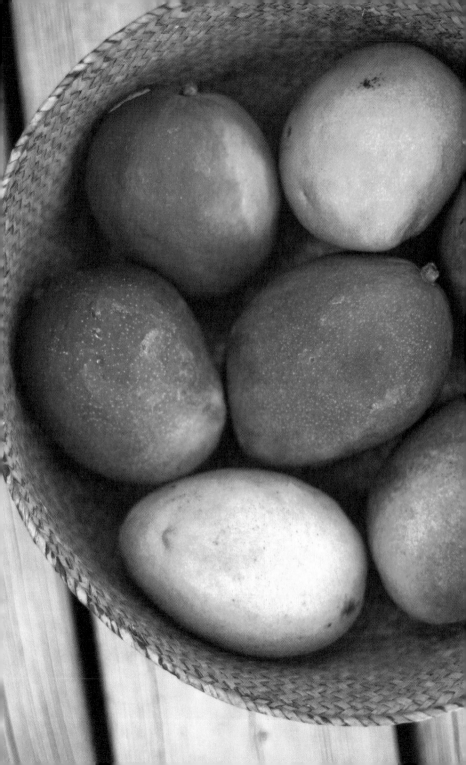

CUCUMBER, PINEAPPLE, AND MANGO

NUTRITIONAL VALUES   85 CALORIES / OG FAT / 1G PROTEIN

21G CARBS / 16G SUGAR / 4MG SODIUM

JUICER TYPE

Cucumber is high in silica, which helps strengthen the connective tissue in skin, making it look more youthful and firm. It also helps gently flush the body of excess water retention, which keeps the skin from looking pallid and puffy. This juice is high in vitamins C and E, two nutrients essential for good skin health.

 1 CUCUMBER
 1 CUP CHOPPED PINEAPPLE
 1 MANGO
 ½ LIME
 3 OR 4 MINT LEAVES (OPTIONAL)

Process all ingredients in your juicer and drink immediately for the best nutritional value. You can also store this juice in an airtight container in the refrigerator for up to 3 days.

PAPAYA POWER

NUTRITIONAL VALUES 80 CALORIES / 0G FAT / 1G PROTEIN

19G CARBS / 13G SUGAR / 10MG SODIUM

JUICER TYPE

This juice's ingredients are great sources of antioxidants, including vitamins C and E and beta-carotene. These nutrients help neutralize free radicals and prevent skin from looking dull, developing wrinkles, and prematurely aging.

1 CUP CHOPPED PAPAYA
1 CUP STRAWBERRIES
½ CUCUMBER
½ LIME

Process all ingredients in your juicer and drink immediately for the best nutritional value. You can also store this juice in an airtight container in the refrigerator for up to 3 days.

COMPLEXION HELPER

NUTRITIONAL VALUES   90 CALORIES / 0G FAT / 2G PROTEIN

21G CARBS / 14G SUGAR / 80MG SODIUM

JUICER TYPE

This juice is a spa day in a glass. Foods rich in vitamins C and E encourage a clear complexion and aid in the reduction of damage from the sun. The high levels of potassium and other minerals also help promote proper hydration and blood health, which are key factors in maintaining your skin's natural healthy glow.

2 APPLES
2 CARROTS
4 OR 5 KALE LEAVES
½ CUP FIRMLY PACKED SPINACH

Process all ingredients in your juicer and drink immediately for the best nutritional value. You can also store this juice in an airtight container in the refrigerator for up to 3 days.

PINEAPPLE–PEPPER–LEMON

NUTRITIONAL VALUES 140 CALORIES / 0G FAT / 1G PROTEIN

32G CARBS / 25G SUGAR / 5MG SODIUM

JUICER TYPE

The mega-antioxidant punch of this juice will slow down your skin's aging process, reducing wrinkles, dry skin, and blemishes. Be sure to include the peels in your juice—they are an incredible source of potassium, calcium, and other minerals essential to firm and healthy skin.

    2 CUPS CHOPPED PINEAPPLE
    1 YELLOW BELL PEPPER
    1 LEMON
    1-INCH PIECE OF GINGER

Process all ingredients in your juicer and drink immediately for the best nutritional value. You can also store this juice in an airtight container in the refrigerator for up to 3 days.

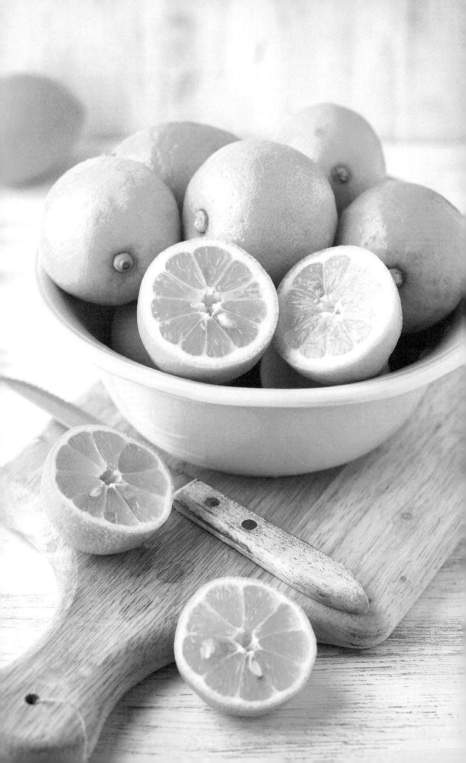

CARROT, PEPPER, AND GINGER

NUTRITIONAL VALUES 95 CALORIES / 1G FAT / 3G PROTEIN

24G CARBS / 15G SUGAR / 70MG SODIUM

JUICER TYPE

Packed with beta-carotene, this juice can help prevent and cure acne and even reduce the symptoms of psoriasis. Ginger's amazing anti-inflammatory properties will also help keep your skin glowing and bright. This juice is also a great source of vitamins E and C, two antioxidants especially important for skin health.

5 CARROTS
1 ORANGE BELL PEPPER
1 PEAR
1–INCH PIECE OF GINGER

Process all ingredients in your juicer and drink immediately for the best nutritional value. You can also store this juice in an airtight container in the refrigerator for up to 3 days.

SKIN-STRENGTHENING ANTIOXIDANT BLAST

NUTRITIONAL VALUES 100 CALORIES / 1G FAT / 1G PROTEIN

23G CARBS / 17G SUGAR / 10MG SODIUM

JUICER TYPE

This superfood-laden juice is packed with vitamins A, B, C, and E, as well as many other antioxidants. These nutrients neutralize free radicals that can damage skin cells and promote premature aging. Yellow beets in particular are a great source of beta-carotene, which helps protect the skin from the sun's rays.

1 YELLOW BEET
1 CUP BLACKBERRIES
1 CUP STRAWBERRIES

Process all ingredients in your juicer and drink immediately for the best nutritional value. You can also store this juice in an airtight container in the refrigerator for up to 3 days.

CUCUMBER, CELERY, AND GREENS SKIN REFRESHER

NUTRITIONAL VALUES   120 CALORIES / 1G FAT / OG PROTEIN

26G CARBS / 18G SUGAR / 5MG SODIUM

JUICER TYPE

This refreshing and tasty juice provides electrolytes, minerals, and antioxidants to help refresh your skin. Cucumber in particular will help bring essential moisture to your skin, while the gentle cleansing properties of the celery and pear will flush your system and help you feel revitalized. For the best flavor, be sure to use a pear that is at its peak ripeness.

> 1 CUCUMBER
> 6 CELERY STALKS
> 1 CUP FIRMLY PACKED SPINACH
> 1 PEAR

Process all ingredients in your juicer and drink immediately for the best nutritional value. You can also store this juice in an airtight container in the refrigerator for up to 3 days.

Silica for silky skin. Silica has been making waves recently for its link to healthy connective tissue as well as healthy hair and nails. The connective tissue in the human body helps keep skin firm and elastic. As we age, this connective tissue loses some of that elasticity, causing wrinkles and sagging skin. Cucumbers and celery are some of the best food sources for natural silica.

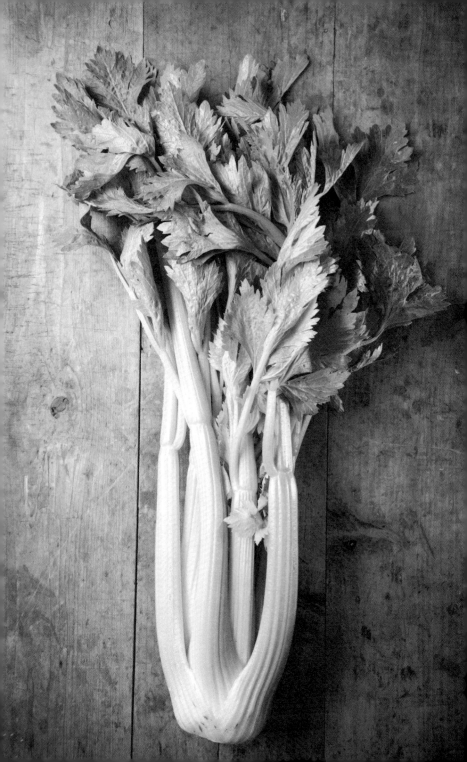

CUCUMBER SKIN CARE

NUTRITIONAL VALUES 120 CALORIES / 1G FAT / 0G PROTEIN

26G CARBS / 14G SUGAR / 5MG SODIUM

JUICER TYPE

Cucumber is filled with silica, a mineral essential for maintaining the body's connective tissue. A diet rich in silica will help promote healthy hair, skin, and nails. This juice is also high in vitamin A, which manages cholesterol levels while improving hair and nail strength.

    1 CUCUMBER
    2 CARROTS
    2 APPLES
    1 CELERY STALK

Process all ingredients in your juicer and drink immediately for the best nutritional value. You can also store this juice in an airtight container in the refrigerator for up to 3 days.

PEACH–STRAWBERRY NECTAR

NUTRITIONAL VALUES 120 CALORIES / 0G FAT / 1G PROTEIN

29G CARBS / 24G SUGAR / 4MG SODIUM

JUICER TYPE

Peaches are a rich source of nutrients. They contain vitamins A, C, E, and K and several minerals, including calcium, copper, iron, magnesium, zinc, manganese, and phosphorus. With that in mind, a peach may be the perfect food for promoting healthy skin. Strawberries and apples are also great sources of skin-healthy antioxidants and will promote healthy hydration.

2 PEACHES
1 CUP STRAWBERRIES
1 APPLE

Process all ingredients in your juicer and drink immediately for the best nutritional value. You can also store this juice in an airtight container in the refrigerator for up to 3 days.

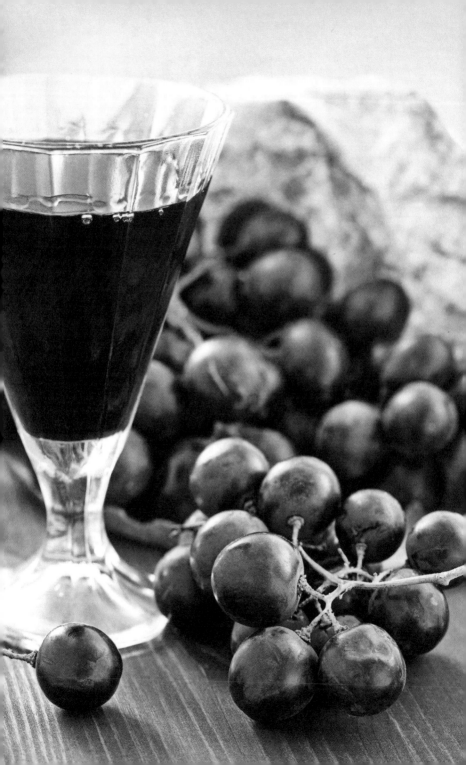

14

KID-FRIENDLY JUICES

GREEN MONSTER

NUTRITIONAL VALUES 60 CALORIES / 0G FAT / 1G PROTEIN

11G CARBS / 7G SUGAR / 30MG SODIUM

JUICER TYPE

Kids will find the bright green color of this juice fun and exciting, and will love the familiar taste of apple juice even more! Choose a larger, sweeter variety of apple such as Fuji for the best flavor result.

2 APPLES
2 CELERY STALKS
3 OR 4 KALE LEAVES

Process all ingredients in your juicer and drink immediately for the best nutritional value. You can also store this juice in an airtight container in the refrigerator for up to 3 days.

CARROT–APPLE

NUTRITIONAL VALUES 70 CALORIES / 0G FAT / 2G PROTEIN

15G CARBS / 6G SUGAR / 35MG SODIUM

JUICER TYPE

Carrot juice is surprisingly sweet and complements apple juice well. This juice is especially tasty when made with tart apples, such as Granny Smith or a freshly picked apple that may not have achieved its full sweetness profile yet. This juice is a tasty way to incorporate a lot of vegetable nutrition into a child's diet.

>   3 OR 4 CARROTS
>   2 APPLES

Process all ingredients in your juicer and drink immediately for the best nutritional value. You can also store this juice in an airtight container in the refrigerator for up to 3 days.

Juicing for a child's health. Any parent can tell you it does no good to prepare healthy foods for your kids if they refuse to eat them. This chapter formulates juices to have that familiar sweet taste kids love. If your child is particularly fussy, feel free to reduce the amount of vegetables in favor of more fruits, gradually shifting more toward the recipe.

SNEAKY VEGETABLE JUICE

NUTRITIONAL VALUES 70 CALORIES / 0G FAT / 1G PROTEIN

16G CARBS / 11G SUGAR / 25MG SODIUM

JUICER TYPE

While the nutrition of fruit juices is great for a growing child, the sugar-laden processed juices found on grocery store shelves leave a lot to be desired. This juice, like many in this chapter, aims to keep the sweet, fruity flavor your kids love, with just enough healthy vegetables to provide a lower-calorie, more nutritious beverage.

2 APPLES
1 CUP FIRMLY PACKED SPINACH
1 YELLOW BEET

Process all ingredients in your juicer and drink immediately for the best nutritional value. You can also store this juice in an airtight container in the refrigerator for up to 3 days.

HEALTHIER APPLE JUICE

NUTRITIONAL VALUES 70 CALORIES / 0G FAT / 2G PROTEIN

17G CARBS / 11G SUGAR / 20MG SODIUM

JUICER TYPE

While apple juice on its own is healthy, it also packs quite a sugar punch. This recipe loads up the juice with added vitamins and minerals while maintaining the sweet apple juice flavor that appeals to kids. You can slowly add more spinach each time your child requests this juice.

3 APPLES
2 CARROTS
½ CUP FIRMLY PACKED SPINACH
   OR OTHER DARK LEAFY GREEN

Process all ingredients in your juicer and drink immediately for the best nutritional value. You can also store this juice in an airtight container in the refrigerator for up to 3 days.

CRANBERRY POWER PUNCH

NUTRITIONAL VALUES 70 CALORIES / 0G FAT / 1G PROTEIN

18G CARBS / 11G SUGAR / 10MG SODIUM

JUICER TYPE

Cranberry juice found in the supermarket often has nearly as much added sugar as soda. This juice takes naturally sweet apples and spikes them with tart, antioxidant-rich cranberries to produce a superfood-spiked juice kids will want to drink. You can also sneak in a small handful of spinach or other leafy greens without anyone being the wiser.

2 APPLES
½ CUP CRANBERRIES
¼ CUP FIRMLY PACKED SPINACH (OPTIONAL)

Process all ingredients in your juicer and drink immediately for the best nutritional value. You can also store this juice in an airtight container in the refrigerator for up to 3 days.

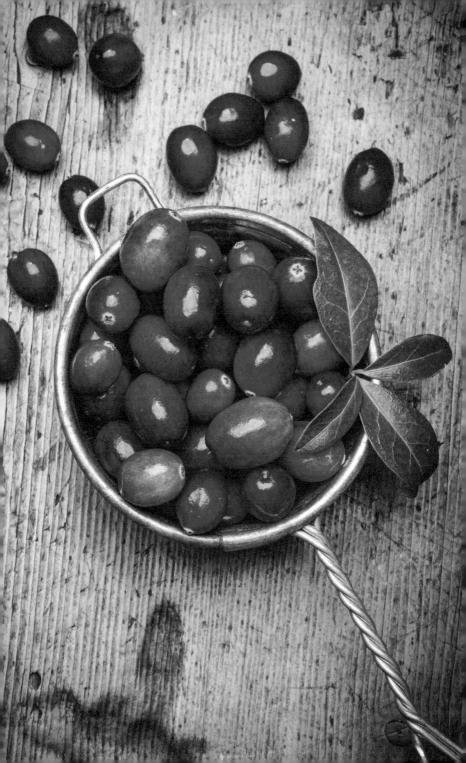

DRINK YOUR VEGETABLES

NUTRITIONAL VALUES 70 CALORIES / 1G FAT / 4G PROTEIN

16G CARBS / 9G SUGAR / 70MG SODIUM

JUICER TYPE

The sweet apple holds its flavor well when combined with these vegetables specifically chosen for their mild or sweet flavors. If your beet still includes the greens, you can use them instead of the kale (or use both if your kids don't mind the extra leafy green flavors).

  1 APPLE
  1 OR 2 CARROTS
  2 KALE LEAVES
  3 ROMAINE LETTUCE LEAVES
  1 SMALL YELLOW BEET

Process all ingredients in your juicer and drink immediately for the best nutritional value. You can also store this juice in an airtight container in the refrigerator for up to 3 days.

When juicing is fun, drinking juice is fun. *Juicers, with their loud whirling mechanisms, can be fascinating for some children. While supervision is absolutely necessary with knives and all appliances, try letting your child help prep the fruits and veggies and even control the portions to an extent. The more ownership they have in making the juice, the more likely they will be to drink it.*

SPROUTS FOR YOUR SPROUT

NUTRITIONAL VALUES   85 CALORIES / 1G FAT / 1G PROTEIN

18G CARBS / 13G SUGAR / 3MG SODIUM

JUICER TYPE

Alfalfa sprouts contain a concentrated amount of vitamins and minerals, including vitamin C, calcium, and vitamin K, yet add only 8 calories—and no fat—per cup. You'll need a masticating or triturating juicer for this one, but once you try this, you may find yourself spiking all your juices with alfalfa sprouts.

1 CUP ALFALFA SPROUTS
1 PEAR
1 CUP STRAWBERRIES
1 APPLE

Process all ingredients in your juicer and drink immediately for the best nutritional value. You can also store this juice in an airtight container in the refrigerator for up to 3 days.

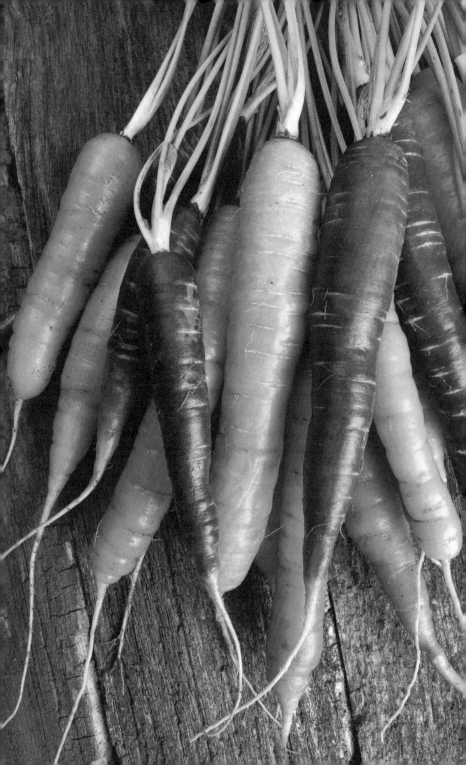

MORNING WAKE-UP CALL

NUTRITIONAL VALUES   80 CALORIES / 0G FAT / 2G PROTEIN

15G CARBS / 8G SUGAR / 55MG SODIUM

JUICER TYPE

This juice complements the high vitamin C and potassium of orange juice with vitamin A–rich carrots. With less sugar and more nutrients than most store-bought juices, this is a great way to start the day for your child.

1 ORANGE
2 CARROTS
1 CELERY STALK
1 APPLE

Process all ingredients in your juicer and drink immediately for the best nutritional value. You can also store this juice in an airtight container in the refrigerator for up to 3 days.

LOWER-CALORIE
GRAPE JUICE

NUTRITIONAL VALUES 120 CALORIES / 0G FAT / 1G PROTEIN

28G CARBS / 27G SUGAR / 15MG SODIUM

JUICER TYPE

Store-bought grape juice is always a favorite—and almost always loaded with sugar. This recipe cuts the sugar by a third while keeping that same delicious flavor. Any of your kid's favorite grapes will work well for this recipe, but red or Concord are two of the best choices. By peeling and seeding the cucumber, you will keep the juice from acquiring too strong of a vegetable flavor, but you can also see if using the whole vegetable will pass muster. To seed, slice the cucumber lengthwise and scoop out the seeds with a teaspoon.

> 2 CUPS RED OR CONCORD GRAPES
> 1 CUCUMBER (PEELED AND SEEDED IF DESIRED)

Process all ingredients in your juicer and drink immediately for the best nutritional value. You can also store this juice in an airtight container in the refrigerator for up to 3 days.

STRAWBERRY–KIWI

NUTRITIONAL VALUES 120 CALORIES / 0G FAT / 1G PROTEIN

30G CARBS / 26G SUGAR / 5MG SODIUM

JUICER TYPE

*Strawberries and kiwi are a combo almost every kid loves. Use
sweet grapes to help cut down on the tartness. To further reduce
any tartness, you can also peel the kiwi. For a special treat, use
frozen berries instead of ice cubes to keep the drink cool.*

    2 CUPS STRAWBERRIES
    2 KIWIS
    1 CUP RED GRAPES

Process all ingredients in your juicer and drink immediately
for the best nutritional value. You can also store this juice in
an airtight container in the refrigerator for up to 3 days.

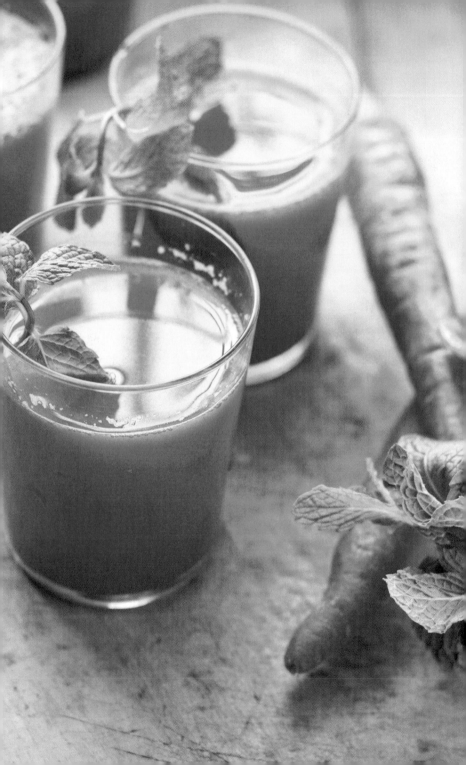

15

LOW-FAT JUICES

DARK AND GREENY

NUTRITIONAL VALUES   60 CALORIES / 0G FAT / 4G PROTEIN

10G CARBS / 5G SUGAR / 10MG SODIUM

JUICER TYPE

This juice provides a great source of complex carbohydrates and proteins, which are especially important when following a low-fat diet. The rich, deep flavors imparted by the beets and spinach will satisfy any cravings for rich foods you might have.

3 KALE LEAVES
1 RED BEET, INCLUDING GREENS
1 CUP FIRMLY PACKED SPINACH
1 CUP CHOPPED BROCCOLI

Process all ingredients in your juicer and drink immediately for the best nutritional value. You can also store this juice in an airtight container in the refrigerator for up to 2 days.

SWEET POTATO AND SPICE

NUTRITIONAL VALUES   60 CALORIES / 0G FAT / 3G PROTEIN

14G CARBS / 8G SUGAR / 30MG SODIUM

JUICER TYPE

Sweet potatoes impart a rich and somewhat starchy quality when juiced, similar to carrots. This juice satisfies cravings for rich desserts while providing a very healthy treat.

> 2 LARGE SWEET POTATOES
> 4 CARROTS
> ½-INCH PIECE OF GINGER
> ½ TEASPOON CINNAMON (OPTIONAL)

Process the first three ingredients in your juicer; stir in the cinnamon if desired. Drink this juice immediately for the best nutritional value, or store in an airtight container in the refrigerator for up to 3 days.

VEGETABLE JUICE

NUTRITIONAL VALUES   70 CALORIES / 0G FAT / 4G PROTEIN

13G CARBS / 4G SUGAR / 70MG SODIUM

JUICER TYPE

This fresh juice closely mimics your favorite store-bought Bloody Mary mix, but with much less salt. This juice will keep well for up to 5 days, so it's a good candidate for making in a larger batch and enjoying all week. Just note that the nutrition levels will be highest when freshly made.

3 TOMATOES

3 CELERY STALKS

2 CARROTS

½ LEMON

2-INCH PIECE OF FRESH HORSERADISH OR 2 TEASPOONS
     PREPARED HORSERADISH (OPTIONAL)

PINCH OF SALT (OPTIONAL)

Process the tomatoes, celery, carrots, lemon, and fresh horse-radish (if using) in your juicer. Stir in the salt and horseradish, if using. Pour the mixture through a fine-mesh sieve into a pitcher for a clearer juice. Drink the juice immediately for the best nutritional value, or store in an airtight container in the refrigerator for up to 5 days.

CELERY AND CARROT

NUTRITIONAL VALUES 70 CALORIES / OG FAT / 3G PROTEIN

14G CARBS / 6G SUGAR / 90MG SODIUM

JUICER TYPE

Celery and carrots complement each other in juice—celery provides a light and aromatic liquid, while carrot juice is rich and sweet. When combined, you get a refreshing and tasty juice that is a great source of vitamins A and C, calcium, and potassium.

3 CELERY STALKS

5 CARROTS

Process all ingredients in your juicer and drink immediately for the best nutritional value. You can also store this juice in an airtight container in the refrigerator for up to 3 days.

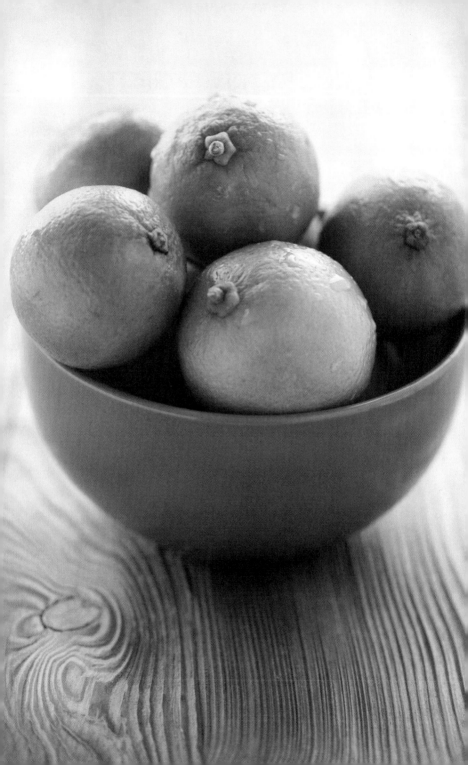

FAT–FIGHTING ZINGY TOMATO JUICE

NUTRITIONAL VALUES   45 CALORIES / OG FAT / 1G PROTEIN

11G CARBS / 9G SUGAR / 30MG SODIUM

JUICER TYPE

In addition to being fat free, the ingredients in this juice help control appetite. Lemon and lime juice in particular have been shown to reduce cravings for fatty foods. Adding a pinch of salt to this juice will bring out the flavor even more.

    4 TOMATOES
    1 LEMON OR 1½ LIMES
    ½–INCH PIECE OF GINGER
    1 JALAPEÑO PEPPER OR OTHER CHILE

Process all ingredients in your juicer and drink immediately for the best nutritional value. You can also store this juice in an airtight container in the refrigerator for up to 3 days.

Fat counters. *All the recipes in this book include basic nutritional information, including the amount of fat. Additionally, you can control a juice's fat content by reducing or eliminating some of the high-fat ingredients, such as avocado and flaxseed oil.*

LOW-FAT GREEN JUICE

NUTRITIONAL VALUES 70 CALORIES / 0G FAT / 1G PROTEIN

18G CARBS / 11G SUGAR / 10MG SODIUM

JUICER TYPE

*In addition to being great for your waistline, this juice also pro-
vides a great source of phytonutrients and cancer-fighting antioxidants. The apple provides a nice shot of vitamin C and some
needed sweetness, so choose a sweeter variety such as Fuji.*

  3 CELERY STALKS
  ½ CUCUMBER
  1 APPLE
  ½ CUP FIRMLY PACKED SPINACH
  3 KALE LEAVES

Process all ingredients in your juicer and drink immediately
for the best nutritional value. You can also store this juice in
an airtight container in the refrigerator for up to 3 days.

*Fat fighters to the rescue. Many foods are so low in calories
that actually more calories are required to process and digest
them than the food provides. Celery, chile peppers, cucumbers,
lemons, limes, garlic, and ginger are foods that help boost the
metabolism without contributing significant calories or fats to
your diet.*

BEET AND CARROT

NUTRITIONAL VALUES   70 CALORIES / 0G FAT / 2G PROTEIN

18G CARBS / 11G SUGAR / 10MG SODIUM

JUICER TYPE

Both beets and carrots are high in magnesium, which helps lower cholesterol. If they look fresh, include the beet greens, which have been shown to promote fat burning in the body and to cleanse the body of surplus fats.

1 OR 2 RED BEETS

4 CARROTS

Process all ingredients in your juicer and drink immediately for the best nutritional value. You can also store this juice in an airtight container in the refrigerator for up to 3 days.

STAR FRUIT AND GREENS

NUTRITIONAL VALUES   75 CALORIES / 0G FAT / 3G PROTEIN

17G CARBS / 11G SUGAR / 20MG SODIUM

JUICER TYPE

High in vitamins C and A, star fruit (also known as carambola) is a great alternative to other fruits when you are looking for something new. The electrolyte-rich juice from cucumbers and romaine lettuce also helps the body maintain proper hydration balance, which can reduce stress-induced food cravings.

> 3 OR 4 STAR FRUIT
> ½ CUCUMBER
> ½ HEAD ROMAINE LETTUCE
> ½ LIME
> 1 APPLE

Process all ingredients in your juicer and drink immediately for the best nutritional value. You can also store this juice in an airtight container in the refrigerator for up to 3 days.

About that star fruit . . . *If you don't have kidney problems, you can eat as much star fruit as you like. But if your kidney function is impaired, do not eat any star fruit. It can result in health complications.*

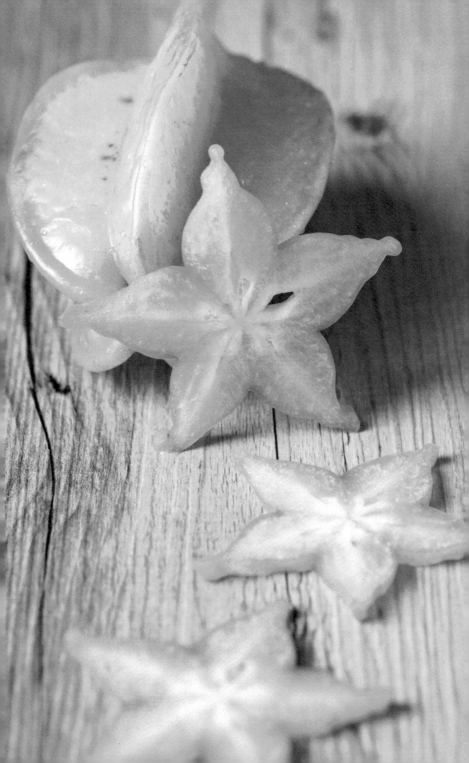

CINNAMON FAT CONTROL

NUTRITIONAL VALUES 100 CALORIES / OG FAT / OG PROTEIN

28G CARBS / 24G SUGAR / 10MG SODIUM

JUICER TYPE

Cinnamon helps regulate blood sugar levels, and research has hinted that it encourages the burning of stored fat. While you can add cinnamon to any juice, apples and blueberries are a particularly great-tasting combination. Cinnamon is also very high in essential minerals and may help lower cholesterol.

2 APPLES
1 CUP BLUEBERRIES
1 TEASPOON CINNAMON

Process the first two ingredients in your juicer; then stir in the cinnamon. Drink the juice immediately for the best nutritional value, or store in an airtight container in the refrigerator for up to 3 days.

CITRUS AND STRAWBERRY

NUTRITIONAL VALUES 110 CALORIES / 0G FAT / 0G PROTEIN

28G CARBS / 20G SUGAR / 4MG SODIUM

JUICER TYPE

Grapefruit is a known appetite suppressant that is also packed with antioxidants. Citrus fruits in general have been shown to curb cravings for fatty foods; they are thought to help increase metabolism and burn fat faster than diets lacking in such fruits.

1 GRAPEFRUIT
1 CUP STRAWBERRIES
1 ORANGE
½ LEMON

Process all ingredients in your juicer and drink immediately for the best nutritional value. You can also store this juice in an airtight container in the refrigerator for up to 3 days.

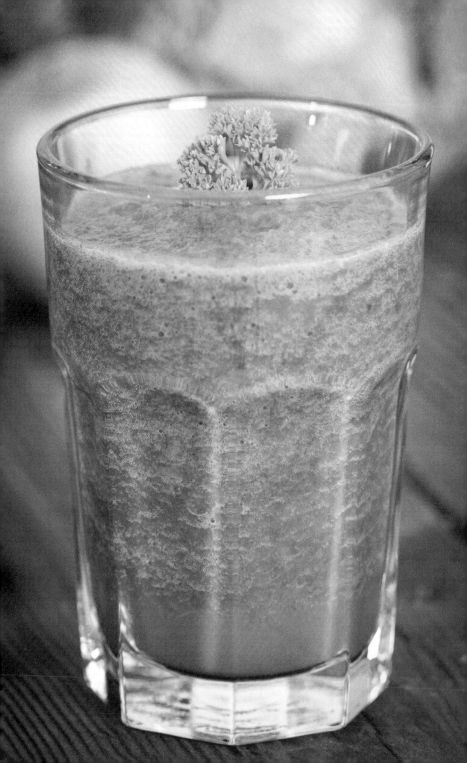

16

PROTEIN
JUICES

ASPARAGUS ZING

NUTRITIONAL VALUES   60 CALORIES / 1G FAT / 8G PROTEIN

9G CARBS / 4G SUGAR / 20MG SODIUM

JUICER TYPE

One of the best juicing ingredients for protein, asparagus is also full of cancer-fighting antioxidants. While pure asparagus juice is actually very tasty on its own, in this recipe, carrots, lime, and cilantro balance its unique flavor. The carrots also add approximately ½ gram of protein each.

8 TO 10 ASPARAGUS SPEARS
2 CARROTS
1 LIME
¼ CUP FIRMLY PACKED CILANTRO

Process all ingredients in your juicer and drink immediately for the best nutritional value. You can also store this juice in an airtight container in the refrigerator for up to 3 days.

ORANGE-BROCCOLI

NUTRITIONAL VALUES 80 CALORIES / 0G FAT / 6G PROTEIN

14G CARBS / 8G SUGAR / 90MG SODIUM

JUICER TYPE

*Ounce for ounce, broccoli juice has more protein than milk!
It does not make the best-tasting juice, however, which is why
you will often find it paired with sweeter and lighter fruits and
veggies. In this recipe, you reap all the benefits of broccoli while
enjoying all the flavor of oranges. Adding cilantro adds a little
extra zing.*

> 2 CUPS CHOPPED BROCCOLI
> 2 ORANGES
> ¼ CUP FIRMLY PACKED CILANTRO (OPTIONAL)

Process all ingredients in your juicer and drink immediately
for the best nutritional value. You can also store this juice in
an airtight container in the refrigerator for up to 2 days.

How much protein is enough? *While some people think
you need a big steak with every dinner to get enough protein, for
most people simply getting about 10 percent of their calories from
high-quality protein is enough. That equates to about 5 grams of
protein in a 100-calorie juice.*

PROTEIN-PACKED
FRUIT JUICE

NUTRITIONAL VALUES 90 CALORIES / 1G FAT / 5G PROTEIN

15G CARBS / 8G SUGAR / 100MG SODIUM

JUICER TYPE

Popeye's food of choice, spinach is not only loaded with iron, but packs a decent protein punch, too. Spinach in general works very well in tart and sweet fruit juices, especially like those found in this juice. So drink your spinach!

> 2 CUPS FIRMLY PACKED SPINACH
> 1 CUP STRAWBERRIES
> 1 GRAPEFRUIT

Process all ingredients in your juicer and drink immediately for the best nutritional value. You can also store this juice in an airtight container in the refrigerator for up to 3 days.

COMPLETE PROTEIN
GREEN JUICE

NUTRITIONAL VALUES 100 CALORIES / 2G FAT / 10G PROTEIN

15G CARBS / 7G SUGAR / 130MG SODIUM

JUICER TYPE

Romaine is not only surprisingly high in protein—it is a complete protein. That means it contains all the amino acids the human body cannot produce on its own. Consuming a wide variety of protein-rich foods, like the ingredients in this juice, helps ensure muscle and overall body health.

1 HEAD ROMAINE LETTUCE
4 CELERY STALKS
1 APPLE
3 ASPARAGUS SPEARS
½ CUCUMBER

Process all ingredients in your juicer and drink immediately for the best nutritional value. You can also store this juice in an airtight container in the refrigerator for up to 3 days.

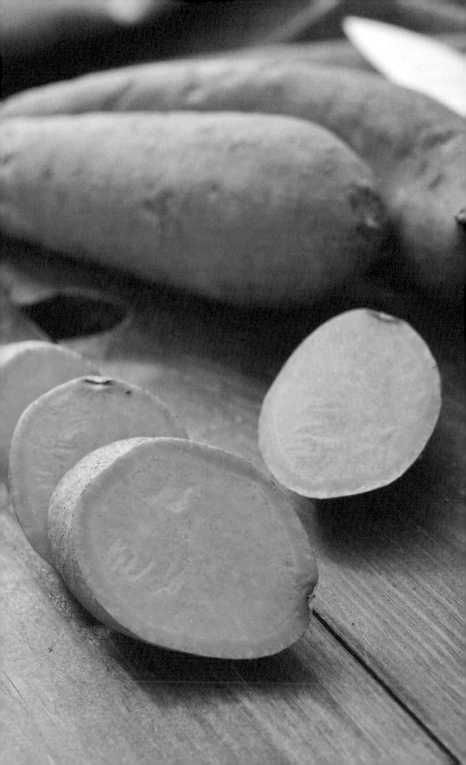

SWEET POTATO AND ASPARAGUS

NUTRITIONAL VALUES   100 CALORIES / 1G FAT / 8G PROTEIN

15G CARBS / 7G SUGAR / 130MG SODIUM

JUICER TYPE

Sweet potatoes, a fantastic source of vitamin A and beta-carotene, also provide a great juice base that's rich in complex carbohydrates, sweet flavor, and more protein than you might expect. Asparagus, packed with as much as a gram of protein per spear, provides the muscle-building amino acids needed for healthy muscle and bones. Adding a bit of lemon helps brighten up this juice while providing a nice vitamin C spike.

> 2 LARGE SWEET POTATOES
> 5 ASPARAGUS SPEARS
> ½ LEMON

Process all ingredients in your juicer and drink immediately for the best nutritional value. You can also store this juice in an airtight container in the refrigerator for up to 3 days.

PROTEIN SPROUT

NUTRITIONAL VALUES 100 CALORIES / 1G FAT / 7G PROTEIN

13G CARBS / 5G SUGAR / 100MG SODIUM

JUICER TYPE

Mung bean sprouts are one of the best plant sources of protein. They also have a pleasantly light and somewhat starchy flavor, which lets you pair them with heavier green juice ingredients. This recipe also includes a tomato, which provides a sweet and tangy flavor as well as additional protein.

    2 CUPS MUNG BEAN SPROUTS
    4 ASPARAGUS SPEARS
    5 KALE LEAVES
    1 TOMATO

Process all ingredients in your juicer and drink immediately for the best nutritional value. You can also store this juice in an airtight container in the refrigerator for up to 3 days.

Complete proteins for complete nutrition. A "complete protein" is a protein that contains all the amino acids the body needs. While all animal proteins fit this description, most plants have only a partial protein profile. The good news is that our bodies are great at storing these amino acids for a fairly long time, so as long as you are getting a varied diet, you don't have to worry too much. If you tend to eat the same foods at every meal, try some of the juices fortified with romaine lettuce, broccoli, bean sprouts, and asparagus to hedge your bet.

HIGH-PROTEIN
VEGETABLE JUICE

NUTRITIONAL VALUES   110 CALORIES / 1G FAT / 11G PROTEIN

16G CARBS / 7G SUGAR / 110MG SODIUM

JUICER TYPE

*One reason romaine isn't well known as a protein source is that in
order to eat an appreciable amount to gain benefit in its non-juice
form, you'd be knocking back several heads of lettuce per day.
Juicing enables you to get the high-quality protein found in this
lettuce quickly and deliciously. This juice compares favorably to
store-bought brands, but is lighter and more aromatic, and has no
added salt.*

> 1 HEAD ROMAINE LETTUCE
> 4 ASPARAGUS SPEARS
> 1 RED BEET
> 3 TO 6 BEET GREEN LEAVES
> 1 CUP CHOPPED BROCCOLI
> ½ CUCUMBER
> 1 TOMATO
> 1 CARROT
> 1 LIME

Process all ingredients in your juicer and drink immediately
for the best nutritional value. You can also store this juice in
an airtight container in the refrigerator for up to 3 days.

APPLE, SPINACH, AND BROCCOLI

NUTRITIONAL VALUES 100 CALORIES / 2G FAT / 10G PROTEIN

15G CARBS / 7G SUGAR / 130MG SODIUM

JUICER TYPE

This very green juice, lightened up with some sweet apples, is a great source of protein. Most dark leafy greens are excellent sources of protein, so feel free to mix and match.

2 APPLES
½ CUP FIRMLY PACKED SPINACH
1 CUP CHOPPED BROCCOLI
2 KALE LEAVES
½ LEMON

Process all ingredients in your juicer and drink immediately for the best nutritional value. You can also store this juice in an airtight container in the refrigerator for up to 2 days.

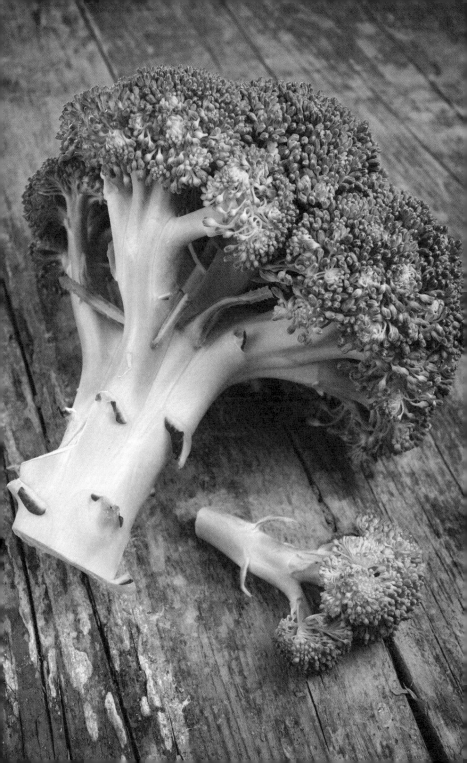

IRON MAN TRAINER

NUTRITIONAL VALUES 120 CALORIES / 2G FAT / 10G PROTEIN

18G CARBS / 7G SUGAR / 140MG SODIUM

JUICER TYPE

*Athletes know that protein is essential for building muscle mass
and maintaining a solid metabolism. This protein-packed juice
is also high in vitamins B and C, which keep you energized while
helping process proteins. You can juice every part of this powerful vegetable, so try to select fresh, local beets with the roots and
greens intact. The very thin roots, which hang from the bottom of
beets, are quite rich in protein.*

8 SMALL RED BEETS, INCLUDING GREENS AND ROOTS
1 CUP FIRMLY PACKED SPINACH
4 ASPARAGUS SPEARS
1 ORANGE

Process all ingredients in your juicer and drink immediately
for the best nutritional value. You can also store this juice in
an airtight container in the refrigerator for up to 3 days.

LEAN, MEAN, AND GREEN

NUTRITIONAL VALUES 160 CALORIES / 2G FAT / 14G PROTEIN

18G CARBS / 7G SUGAR / 180MG SODIUM

JUICER TYPE

Many gardeners love growing broccoli and cauliflower, but generally eat only the heads, leaving the stems for the compost pile. Feel free to use just the stalks in your juicer. While not quite as nutritious as cauliflower and broccoli heads, the stalks are still incredibly healthful and carry a lighter flavor.

1 CUP CHOPPED BROCCOLI
1 CUP CHOPPED CAULIFLOWER
3 COLLARD GREEN LEAVES
1 HEAD ROMAINE LETTUCE
1 LIME

Process all ingredients in your juicer and drink immediately for the best nutritional value. You can also store this juice in an airtight container in the refrigerator for up to 2 days.

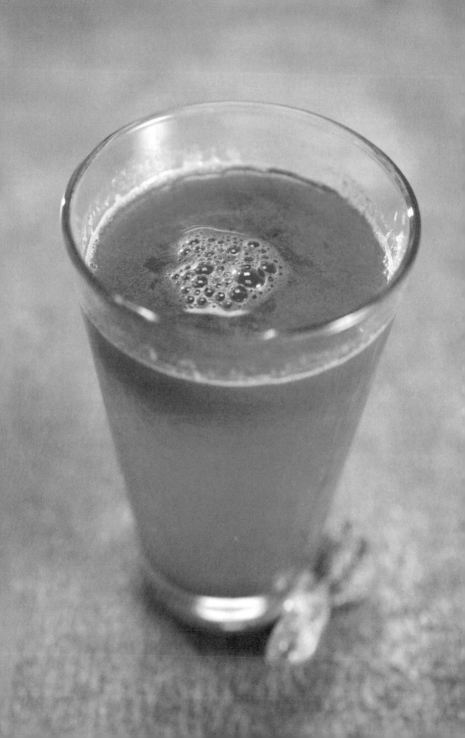

17

WEIGHT-LOSS
JUICES

CUCUMBER–MINT–LEMON

NUTRITIONAL VALUES   45 CALORIES / 0G FAT / 2G PROTEIN

10G CARBS / 5G SUGAR / 6MG SODIUM

JUICER TYPE

The biggest draw of cucumbers as part of a weight-loss diet is their low calorie count. However, the benefits don't stop there. Cucumbers are also rich sources of electrolytes, especially potassium, which help reduce water retention associated with excess salt in the diet. They also provide a good source of fiber, which helps keep you feeling full all day.

2 CUCUMBERS
¼ CUP FIRMLY PACKED MINT LEAVES
½ LEMON

Process all ingredients in your juicer and drink immediately for the best nutritional value. You can also store this juice in an airtight container in the refrigerator for up to 3 days.

CANTALOUPE–GINGER

NUTRITIONAL VALUES 80 CALORIES / 1G FAT / 0G PROTEIN

19G CARBS / 17G SUGAR / 16MG SODIUM

JUICER TYPE

Cantaloupe is surprisingly low in calories, despite its sweet taste. It also packs in the nutrients, including omega-3 healthy fats, vitamin C, vitamin A, and potassium. Additionally, even juiced, cantaloupe provides a great source of fiber that will help you stay regular and feel full.

2 CUPS CHOPPED CANTALOUPE
½-INCH PIECE OF GINGER

Process all ingredients in your juicer and drink immediately for the best nutritional value. You can also store this juice in an airtight container in the refrigerator for up to 3 days.

METABOLISM BOOST

NUTRITIONAL VALUES 70 CALORIES / 1G FAT / 2G PROTEIN

14G CARBS / 12G SUGAR / 15MG SODIUM

JUICER TYPE

All the ingredients in this juice will power up your metabolism, helping you burn more calories throughout the day. Feel free to double up on the broccoli, and remove the asparagus if you want to use only local in-season produce. In addition to its metabolism-boosting properties, this cleansing juice will keep you feeling fresh and alert. Dark-skinned grapes (such as Concord) are optimal in this recipe, but any grape will work.

½ CUP CHOPPED BROCCOLI
2 ASPARAGUS SPEARS
½ CUP FIRMLY PACKED WATERCRESS
2 KALE LEAVES
1 CUP GRAPES

Process all ingredients in your juicer and drink immediately for the best nutritional value. You can also store this juice in an airtight container in the refrigerator for up to 2 days.

Benefits of a strong metabolism. *Developing a strong metabolism benefits more than your waistline. A strong metabolism will give you more energy throughout the day, increases brainpower, and can help manage depression and anxiety. Sleep, proper nutrition, exercise, and a low-stress lifestyle are the keys to keeping your metabolism high.*

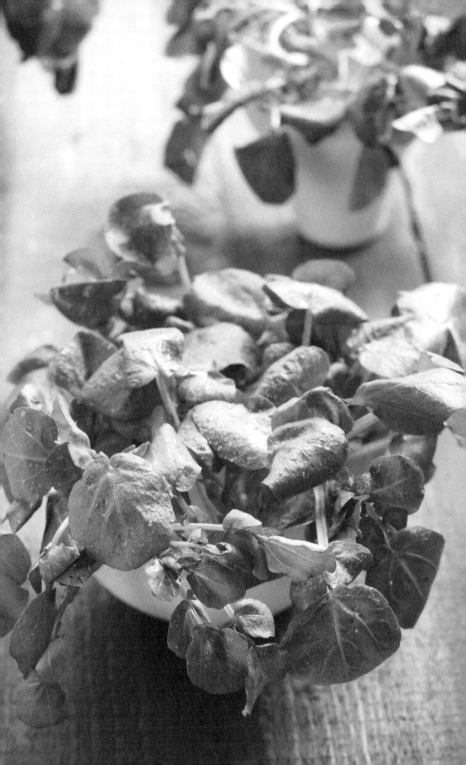

WATERMELON, BROCCOLI, AND APPLE

NUTRITIONAL VALUES   90 CALORIES / OG FAT / 3G PROTEIN

19G CARBS / 11G SUGAR / 15MG SODIUM

JUICER TYPE

This juice works well if you're just starting to incorporate juice into your weight-loss regimen. With a high level of electrolytes, this juice replenishes the body after intense workouts. You can also drink this juice before a workout to stay hydrated and energized. Additionally, the watercress acts as a mild diuretic and digestive cleanser, which aids weight loss.

    1 APPLE
    1 CUP CHOPPED WATERMELON
    1 CUP CHOPPED BROCCOLI
    ½ CUP FIRMLY PACKED WATERCRESS

Process all ingredients in your juicer and drink immediately for the best nutritional value. You can also store this juice in an airtight container in the refrigerator for up to 2 days.

APPETITE-CONTROLLING GRAPEFRUIT AND LEMON

NUTRITIONAL VALUES   90 CALORIES / 1G FAT / 1G PROTEIN

22G CARBS / 14G SUGAR / 3MG SODIUM

JUICER TYPE

Grapefruit and lemon are both well-known appetite suppressants. One study showed that people who ate half a grapefruit with each meal for a month lost 3.6 pounds compared to the control group. While grapefruit is the king among citrus in this area, all citrus offer some benefit as well, so feel free to mix things up a little. Choose a lower-acid Meyer lemon if the acidity of this juice is too much.

 1 GRAPEFRUIT
 1 LEMON

Process both ingredients in your juicer and drink immediately for the best nutritional value. You can also store this juice in an airtight container in the refrigerator for up to 3 days.

MANGO–CANTALOUPE

NUTRITIONAL VALUES 120 CALORIES / 0G FAT / 4G PROTEIN

29G CARBS / 27G SUGAR / 37MG SODIUM

JUICER TYPE

The main ingredients in this juice provide all the vitamins A and C you'll need for the day. Despite being almost sinfully sweet, this juice has half the calories of most store-bought juices (not to mention much more nutritional value). Both the mango and cantaloupe contain easily accessible sugars and electrolytes that can turbocharge your energy level, making this particular recipe fantastic fuel for cardio training.

1 MANGO, CHOPPED
2 CUPS CHOPPED CANTALOUPE
½ CUCUMBER

Process all ingredients in your juicer and drink immediately for the best nutritional value. You can also store this juice in an airtight container in the refrigerator for up to 3 days.

PINEAPPLE, CUCUMBER, AND ROMAINE

NUTRITIONAL VALUES   150 CALORIES / 1G FAT / 7G PROTEIN

35G CARBS / 25G SUGAR / 5MG SODIUM

JUICER TYPE

Pineapple is another fruit with well-known appetite-suppressing properties, while also being decadently sweet. Cucumber and romaine both provide protein and filling fiber, making this juice a great low-calorie meal replacement.

  2 CUPS CHOPPED PINEAPPLE
  ½ CUCUMBER
  ½ HEAD ROMAINE LETTUCE

Process all ingredients in your juicer and drink immediately for the best nutritional value. You can also store this juice in an airtight container in the refrigerator for up to 3 days.

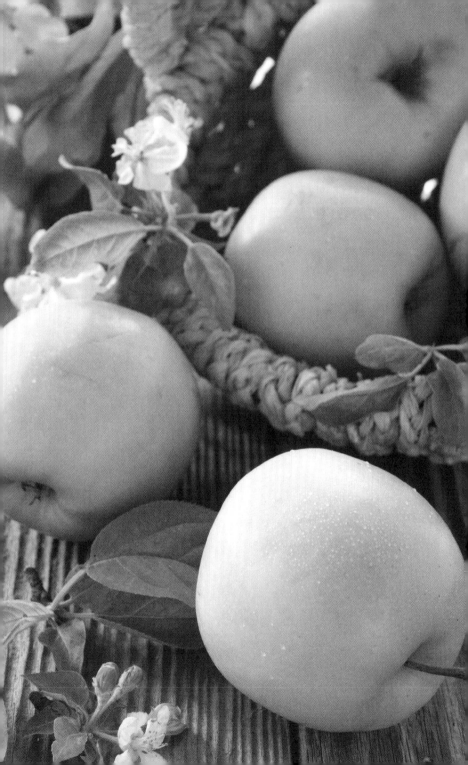

WEIGHT-LOSS
MASTER JUICE

NUTRITIONAL VALUES   100 CALORIES / 2G FAT / 5G PROTEIN

19G CARBS / 11G SUGAR / 2MG SODIUM

JUICER TYPE

This juice combines several ingredients that tackle hunger, speed metabolism, and aid in weight loss. The romaine lettuce supply a complete, satiating protein, while acting as mild diuretics to prevent water retention. The spinach, in addition to packing a major nutrient punch, is also loaded with chlorophyll, which helps cleanse the body. Cayenne pepper helps boost the metabolism, while the optional spirulina and psyllium additives both help suppress appetite and aid in feeling full.

½ HEAD ROMAINE LETTUCE
1 CUP FIRMLY PACKED SPINACH
1 APPLE
1 TEASPOON CAYENNE PEPPER
1 TEASPOON SPIRULINA (OPTIONAL)
1 TEASPOON PSYLLIUM (OPTIONAL)

Process the romaine, spinach, and apple in your juicer; then stir in the cayenne and the spirulina and psyllium if desired. Drink this juice immediately for the best nutritional value, or store in an airtight container in the refrigerator for up to 3 days.

VEGETABLE WEIGHT–LOSS JUICE

NUTRITIONAL VALUES 150 CALORIES / 2G FAT / 4G PROTEIN

30G CARBS / 10G SUGAR / 35MG SODIUM

JUICER TYPE

This juice is like a salad in a glass, providing nutrients, fiber, and energy to get you through a challenging weight-loss day. The watercress helps cleanse your digestive system and prevents water retention. The leafy greens supply a megadose of nutrients and fiber to keep you energized and full. The tomatoes, cucumber, and apple also help suppress appetite while giving you the electrolytes and energy needed to fuel workouts.

2 TOMATOES
½ CUCUMBER
1 CELERY STALK
½ CUP FIRMLY PACKED SPINACH
2 KALE LEAVES
½ CUP FIRMLY PACKED WATERCRESS
1 APPLE
3 PITTED DATES (OPTIONAL)

Process all ingredients in your juicer and drink immediately for the best nutritional value. You can also store this juice in an airtight container in the refrigerator for up to 3 days.

BANANA–STRAWBERRY–APPLE SHAKE

NUTRITIONAL VALUES 200 CALORIES / 1G FAT / 2G PROTEIN

46G CARBS / 34G SUGAR / 2MG SODIUM

JUICER TYPE

This juice, which requires a blender, makes a delicious, filling breakfast that comes in at 200 calories. Bananas are high in fiber and potassium, and they keep you full for hours. Strawberries and apples provide a low-calorie sweetness that also helps cleanse your system of toxins and excess water retention. Feel free to add some nonfat yogurt to the blender for a little extra protein and calcium.

    1 CUP STRAWBERRIES
    1 APPLE
    1 BANANA
    ¼–½ CUP NONFAT YOGURT (OPTIONAL)

Process the strawberries and apple in your juicer; transfer the juice to a blender. Add the banana and process until smooth. Add nonfat yogurt, if desired. Drink immediately.

Bananas for weight loss. *Some people look at the relatively high calories and sugar in a banana and think it should play no role in a weight-loss diet. However, nothing could be further from the truth! Bananas are high in fiber and essential nutrients that can help you feel full longer. Additionally, the high levels of potassium and other electrolytes help flush the body of excess water that can contribute to bloating.*

FRUIT AND VEGETABLE NUTRITION CHARTS

FRUITS FOR JUICING *Serving size = 100 grams*

Food	Calories	Protein (g)	Carbs (g)	Fats (g)	Fiber (g)
Apple	50	0.26	13.8	0.17	2.4
Apricot	48	1.00	11.0	0.00	2.0
Blackberries	43	1.39	9.6	0.49	5.3
Blood orange	50	0.00	11.0	0.00	2.0
Blueberries	57	0.74	14.5	0.33	2.4
Cantaloupe	34	0.84	8.6	0.19	0.9
Cherries	50	1.00	12.2	0.30	1.6
Cranberries	46	0.00	12.0	0.00	5.0
Figs	74	1.00	19.0	0.00	3.0
Gooseberries	44	1.00	10.0	1.00	4.0
Grapes	69	0.72	18.0	0.16	0.9
Grapefruit	42	0.77	10.7	0.14	1.7
Guava	68	3.00	14.0	1.00	5.0 ➤

➤ FRUITS FOR JUICING   *Serving size = 100 grams*

Food	Calories	Protein (g)	Carbs (g)	Fats (g)	Fiber (g)
Honeydew	36	1.00	9.0	0.00	1.0
Jicama	38	1.00	9.0	0.00	5.0
Kiwi	61	1.00	14.6	0.52	3.0
Kumquat	71	2.00	16.0	1.00	6.0
Lemon	29	1.10	9.3	0.30	2.8
Lime	30	1.00	11.0	0.00	3.0
Mango	70	0.50	17.0	0.27	1.8
Nectarine	44	1.00	11.0	0.00	2.0
Orange	47	0.94	11.7	0.12	2.4
Papaya	39	0.61	9.8	0.14	1.8
Passion fruit	97	2.20	23.4	0.70	10.4
Peach	39	0.91	9.5	0.25	1.5
Pear	58	0.38	13.8	0.12	3.1
Persimmon	127	1.00	33.0	0.00	0.0
Pineapple	50	0.54	13.5	0.12	1.4
Plum	46	1.00	11.0	0.00	1.0
Pomegranate	83	1.67	18.7	1.17	4.0
Raspberries	52	1.20	11.9	0.65	6.5
Star fruit	31	1.00	7.0	0.00	3.0
Strawberries	32	0.67	7.7	0.30	2.0
Tangerine	53	0.81	13.3	0.31	1.8
Watermelon	30	1.00	8.0	0.00	0.0

VEGETABLES FOR JUICING *Serving size = 100 grams*

Food	Calories	Protein (g)	Carbs (g)	Fats (g)	Fiber (g)
Arugula	25	2.58	3.65	0.66	1.6
Asparagus	20	2.20	3.38	0.12	2.1
Beets	45	1.61	9.56	0.17	2.8
Bell pepper	31	0.99	6.03	0.30	2.1
Bok choy	13	1.50	2.18	0.20	1.0
Broccoli	34	2.82	6.64	0.37	2.6
Brussels sprouts	43	3.38	8.95	0.30	3.8
Cabbage	25	1.30	5.80	0.10	2.5
Carrots	41	0.93	9.58	0.24	2.8
Cauliflower	25	1.92	4.97	0.28	2.0
Celeriac	42	1.00	9.00	0.00	2.0
Celery	16	1.00	3.00	0.00	2.0
Collard greens	30	2.45	5.69	0.42	3.6
Cucumber	15	0.65	3.63	0.11	0.5
Dandelion greens	45	3.00	9.00	1.00	4.0
Kale	50	3.30	10.00	0.70	2.0
Kohlrabi	27	2.00	6.00	0.00	4.0
Mustard greens	26	3.00	5.00	0.00	3.0
Onion	40	1.00	9.00	0.00	2.0
Parsnips	75	1.20	18.00	0.30	4.9 ➤

Food	Calories	Protein (g)	Carbs (g)	Fats (g)	Fiber (g)
Pumpkin	26	1.00	6.50	0.10	0.5
Radishes	16	1.00	3.00	0.00	2.0
Romaine lettuce	15	1.36	2.79	0.15	1.3
Rutabaga	36	1.00	8.00	0.00	3.0
Scallions	32	2.00	7.00	0.00	3.0
Spinach	23	2.86	3.63	0.39	2.2
Sugar snap peas	42	3.00	8.00	0.00	3.0
Summer squash	16	1.00	3.00	0.00	1.0
Sweet potato	86	1.60	20.10	0.05	3.0
Swiss chard	19	3.27	3.74	0.20	1.6
Tomatoes	18	0.90	3.90	0.20	1.8
Turnip	32	1.00	7.00	0.00	3.0
Turnip greens	32	1.00	7.00	0.00	3.0
Wheatgrass	23	2.00	3.00	0.00	0.0

RECIPE INDEX

INDEX